ENDOR

"In SOUL HEALTH, Dr. Katherine Kelly restores the concept of the soul to its rightful place in our lives. This important book will give anyone insight into a more fruitful, fulfilling life."

~~ Larry Dossey, MD
Author of *Recovering the Soul* and *The Power of Premonitions*

"SOUL HEALTH is a thoughtful, practical guide to regaining balance and creating a truly fulfilling life. Dr. Kelly is a pioneer and her Soul Health Model is a complete look at health, healing, and cultivating the true soul's expression. The tools she offers can be used by anyone to gain a deeper understanding of their human condition and their soul's evolution."

~~ Sarah McLean, Director of the McLean Meditation Institute
Best-Selling author of *Soul-Centered:*
Transform Your Life in 8 Weeks with Meditation

"In SOUL HEALTH, Dr. Kelly has chosen an ancient archetype, the tree, as scaffolding for teaching a fresh and original model for creating a balanced life in harmony with one's soul. Her own tap roots run deep in the earth as an experienced therapist, teacher, scholar, intuitive and spiritual seeker. With each branch she examines another aspect of living, each requiring balance in the outer world while taking direction from the soul and in turn feeding soul intention by choices made in the world. The book is rich with wise insights, provocative exercises, and probing questions for the reader. This is truly a growth manual and a personal bedside book that one will return to over and over with highlighter in hand."

~~ Gloria Karpinski, Interfaith Minister
Author of *Where Two Worlds Touch* and *Barefoot on Holy Ground*

"SOUL HEALTH is a book to keep at your bedside and on your desk as a daily reference—one you will want to read and refer to over and over again. It will help your patients, but it will also help your own soul. Dr. Katherine Kelly's book is a guide to being optimally healthy for those who have lost their way and also those who think they are "just fine.""

~~ Elizabeth Davis, MD, General Psychiatry

"SOUL HEALTH is a must read not only for therapists but for anyone who needs a thought-provoking and practical guide to enhance their lives. Dr. Kelly has significantly transformed the way we understand and utilize our soul. Through her newly-developed model of aligning with spirit, we now have a way to truly live a life filled with radiant health."

~~ Cheryl Rubin, MSW, LCSW, Clinical Social Worker

"I love SOUL HEALTH!!! Dr. Kelly asks wonderful questions that make you think and go deep within. This book is a great tool in our own personal evolution."

~~ Lynn A. Hawks, Energy Therapist and Interfaith Minister

SOUL HEALTH

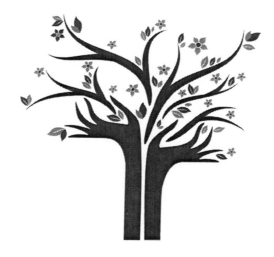

SOUL HEALTH

ALIGNING WITH SPIRIT FOR RADIANT LIVING

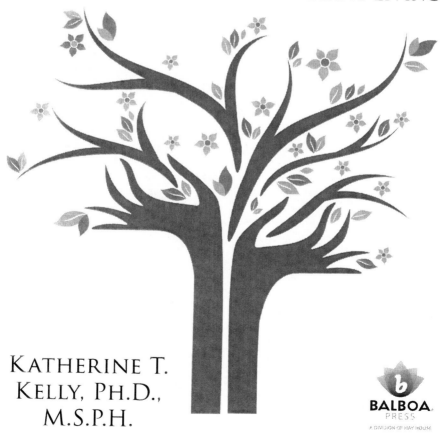

KATHERINE T.
KELLY, Ph.D.,
M.S.P.H.

BALBOA
PRESS
A DIVISION OF HAY HOUSE

Balboa Press books may be ordered through booksellers or by contacting:

Balboa Press
A Division of Hay House
1663 Liberty Drive
Bloomington, IN 47403
www.balboapress.com
1-(877) 407-4847

Printed in the United States of America

ISBN: 978-1-4525-6562-0 (sc)
ISBN: 978-1-4525-6564-4 (hc)
ISBN: 978-1-4525-6563-7 (e)

Library of Congress Control Number: 2012923674

Balboa Press rev. date: 1/30/2013

To the Human Condition

*In the attitude of silence the soul finds the path in
a clearer light, and what is elusive and deceptive
resolves itself into crystal clearness.*

~~ Mahatma Gandhi

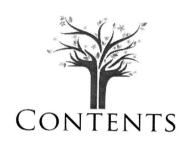

CONTENTS

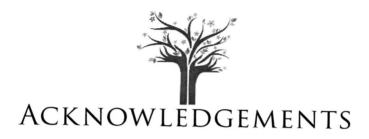

ACKNOWLEDGEMENTS

The premise of this book is that all aspects of daily life—our human condition—affect our ability to reach radiant health and, as a result, also affect our soul's evolution. How, then, does one acknowledge and thank every soul who contributed to the evolution of this book?

I credit each and every soul whose path I've crossed throughout my own evolution as a human, a psychologist, and a soul. I offer my deep gratitude to the many authors, teachers, and spiritual leaders, whether in this world or beyond, whose wisdom has allowed me to advance the evolution of others, and has most certainly challenged me to evolve during my own journey within the human condition.

I am most indebted to the thousands of clients and workshop participants I have had the privilege to know and assist throughout their healing journeys. There is nothing more rewarding than growing souls, and I am truly honored to have shared both your trials and successes on your path to healing. You continue to be my most valued and wisest teachers.

I am also blessed with many who have played supportive roles in my personal soul journey. I extend special thanks to my long-time friend, Stacy Ruskin, who has witnessed me wrestle with the human condition more than anyone. There are no words to fully express my gratitude for your unwavering support throughout the last 28 years. You have witnessed me wrestle with the human condition more than anyone, and yet, you continue to laugh with me, cry with me, and most importantly, remain patient with me in all of my endeavors toward soul growth. You are my soul sister, and I am forever grateful.

To my father who made his transition so long ago—thank you for supporting all of my various aspirations from such an early age. Even from beyond, I have no doubt that you have overseen the writing of this book.

To my mother, siblings, dear friends, and colleagues—I extend my deep gratitude for your support, curiosity, understanding, and patience throughout this process. Without you, I would not be who I am, nor would The Soul Health Model exist.

Several other soul supporters warrant recognition. Lynn Hawks, Cheryl Rubin, Melissa Hassard, and Carol Walsh deserve special thanks as they reviewed the manuscript in its various stages and served as my alternate "eyes" as the final words emerged. Your honest feedback not only urged me forward, but also made this book "whole." Thank you.

Very special thanks go to Chara Murray, the visionary graphic artist who helped me to pictorially capture The Soul Health Model. I remain in awe of your ability to merge my ideas into such a marvelous depiction of radiant health after only a brief conversation. You are truly a gifted soul!

I am indebted to my editor, Kate Maloy, for her tremendous

mastery of the English language and for her assistance in refining the ideas offered here. As a writer I expected to benefit from your grammatical expertise; what I received was unforeseen edification—a solidifying and enhancement of my thoughts as well as an acceleration of my evolution as an author. For this, I am eternally grateful.

I hold deep gratitude for authors Larry Dossey, M.D., Gloria Karpinski, and Sarah McLean, who provided such kind words of support for *Soul Health*. My thanks also go to Cheryl Rubin, MSW, LCSW, Elizabeth Davis, M.D., and Lynn Hawks, Energy Therapist and Interfaith Minister, for both your support and endorsement of this literary endeavor. Your interest and encouragement will never be forgotten.

And finally, to Morton and Chloe, the most patient and precious angel dogs in the world. I am blessed by your presence.

SOUL HEALTH

ALIGNING WITH SPIRIT FOR RADIANT LIVING

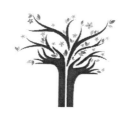

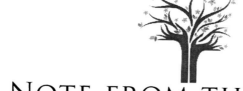

A NOTE FROM THE AUTHOR

Soul Health: Aligning with Spirit for Radiant Living is intended as a user-friendly conceptual model for attaining the deepest and most complete form of health, which is soul health. As you will see, soul health is multidimensional, and this book is certain both to expand and to deepen your awareness of what may be missing from your life, even as it gives you the conceptual tools for radiant living. *Soul Health* is also a guide for your soul's evolution, which becomes possible only when you provide the elements essential to its growth.

This book can be your instructional guide and workbook on your path to soul health. Throughout the chapters, you will find many questions to answer, thoughts to ponder, and exercises to explore. I encourage you to take your time reading the chapters and assessing the state of your soul; that is the best way to fully assimilate the information offered. I also highly recommend that you purchase a notebook or journal in which to record your own thoughts, ideas, and actions in response to everything this book covers. Feel free to highlight the book itself, make notes in the margins, and dog-ear important pages as you read the chapters. Those who participate in this active way tend not only to gain the most out of their reading, but also to invest the most in developing their own soulful approaches to life. Documenting your journey will be a useful tool as you discover your soul and learn how to nurture its radiant health.

Although the overall concept of soul health is new to many people, this book presents it in a way that will stimulate thinking, but not overwhelm you. As you read through this book and complete the exercises provided, make sure you recognize what is already working for you along with what you would like to change or enhance as you envision your optimal soul health. This book allows you to be flexible in integrating the ideas and techniques. It should help you experience a heightened awareness just by reading it, but it should also ignite your desire to make active use of its suggestions and tools.

Most of all, understand that your soul health is a journey—one in which you can learn and grow as well as one that is enjoyable. Radiant living may take some work, but the pay-off is optimal soul health.

Through the blessings of my own journey, it is no accident that I share *Soul Health* with you now—in this time of expanding consciousness. May your journey lead the way to many rich experiences within the human condition as you continue your path to radiant health—and ultimately to your soul's evolution.

In Shared Light,

Katherine T. Kelly, Ph.D., M.S.P.H.

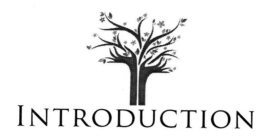

INTRODUCTION

SOUL HEALTH:
THE CORE OF RADIANT LIVING

If we dwell in spirit, or Soul, we are living in happiness,
for Soul is a happy entity. ~~ Paul Twitchell

To know your soul is to know true health. Only then can you reach radiant living. But most people find it hard to manage the common cold gracefully, let alone to live a fully soulful and radiant life.

So, what is missing? What keeps you from feeling a complete sense of health and well-being? What is not quite right in your world? Perhaps more importantly, how do you know that something is missing or off track when you don't even know what that "something" is?

The primary void in our modern approach to health is any concern for our soul. Unlike early conceptualizations of health, our current ones lend very little, if any, value to the influence of our soul on our everyday lives. As a result, we are not only losing contact with our most vital ally, but also losing track of what it means to experience optimal health.

The soul is at the hub of all aspects of our health and well-being. It is the nucleus of every action, behavior, thought, emotion, ache or pain, and it houses an inherent wisdom about what we want and need for optimal vitality. Each discomfort—or "symptom of the soul"— alerts us that something is amiss. This *dis*-ease is our soul's attempt to warn us that our lives are somehow misaligned with the needs of our innermost core and that if we leave it unattended, we will suffer in one way or another. We will fail to reach radiant health.

Our soul's most natural state is that of unimpeded growth. Therefore, our soul's evolution depends entirely on our willingness and ability to balance our lives in such a way that we create an unobstructed environment for its growth. Unfortunately, our day-to-day challenges— our inherent human condition—inevitably gets in the way. Modern healthcare models fail to include a *Soul Health* approach; they generally only focus on physical aspects of our well-being. And despite the fact that doctor-patient relationship research indicates that over 90 percent of those seeking medical care would like their provider to integrate a spiritual component in their healing, this vital element still remains unaddressed.

Early in my training as a psychologist I came across the National Wellness Institute's model of "wellness." The model included six components of health—physical, psychological, social, environmental, intellectual and spiritual—which, when balanced, lead a person to find their fullest potential or their highest achieved sense of feeling "well." Although this model was not included in my formal education, I immediately started conceptualizing my clinical work from this perspective. The model took my clinical work far beyond the typical "bio-psycho-social" model that I was taught and allowed me to expand my understanding of what was and wasn't working in my clients' lives— not to mention my own. It just made sense.

After I completed my training, I continued to use the model not only in my psychotherapy work, but also in my teaching in medical school systems, corporate health environments, and public venues. Over time, I realized there were key components of everyday life that were missing or little acknowledged in the model—ones that couldn't be ignored in the quest for a person's optimal wellness. So, after opening a holistic health and wellness center of my own, the model evolved into what I called the *Whole Health Model*. I used the metaphor of a tree to explain the "branches of health" (hence the name of my center— *Branches Holistic Health and Wellness Center*). The three branches I then added to the original six were Financial, Interpersonal, and Sexual Health. It was obvious to me that these additional elements played a major role in understanding an overall sense of "wellness" or "whole health." I offered the model to clients and professionals as an educational tool to help them understand the interconnectedness of all the branches and it proved quite effective in helping people re-conceptualize their approach to healing.

Ironically, although my *Whole Health Model* was created to represent the branches of health in which I offered services through my center, it also offered the stimulus that helped me decide to close it. At the time, I had fourteen employees (psychotherapists, a nutritionist/chef, massage therapist, energy therapist, fitness trainers, and yoga and tai chi instructors) housed in a 10,000 square foot building where we offered a variety of health services. While the clients' wellness was improving, my own was failing. And because I have always striven to be a good role model for clients, it became clear that I could not do that as long as I remained the owner of the business. I knew I couldn't practice what I preached, which was not good enough for me. I also knew I would not be able to dedicate the time I needed to my writing since I had sat down to my computer only three times in the four years I owned the center.

I maintained my psychotherapy practice throughout that difficult time but I was exhausted and unbalanced in many ways— which lent validity to the *Whole Health Model*. It took me nearly two years to fully recover from that adventure, but all was not lost. During this time, I was finally able to recognize two key elements in the most recent evolution of the model—both of which were strikingly obvious once I saw them.

First, in talking to a client, I suddenly saw another missing branch, which was Recreational Health (i.e., Fun and Leisure). Although the creation of *Branches* had been a great deal of fun, the maintenance of it was not. Most definitely, there is no leisure in owning a business like that. Multiple studies show the positive health benefits of fun and laughter, but for some reason, it hadn't crossed my mind to include this as a branch of health. The reason must be obvious—like many, I was just too busy to think of it or include enough of it in my own life. Regardless, that new branch rounded out the rest of the tree and breathed obvious life into the overall model.

However, the most striking omission to the model was the soul. Although it is impossible to fully define, each of us has an inherent wisdom about what we want and need in life in order to experience our most fulfilled level of well-being— our *radiant vitality*. We each know what makes us feel alive and what dims or deadens our psyche. Somehow we know our own radiance and we know when we are *living* instead of just *existing*. This inherent wisdom stems from our soul—the core of both who we are and who we are meant to be if we allow it. If given the chance, our soul will serve as our most vital ally.

Our soul is an entity of its own. It yearns to grow and evolve despite the conditions we place it in. If left to its own devices, it will joyfully create its own expansive inertia. As a result, our soul will continue along the path of infinite growth. Scientists have said that the human body has evolved as much as it is going to. But our inner core—our soul—has infinite potential to evolve, to shine and ultimately glow. The challenge is that we must learn to work in tandem with our human side—our human condition—and our most vital ally, our soul, in order to achieve our most radiant vitality. And only then do we set the stage for unimpeded growth and evolution.

What I once called the *Whole Health Model* thus evolved into the *Soul Health Model.* As you will read, the ten essential elements of the human condition (Physical, Psychological, Social, Interpersonal, Intellectual, Financial, Environmental, Spiritual, Sexual, and Recreational) are the keys to balancing our everyday lives; they are the essential ingredients for creating our optimal health. And it is the complex interplay among these elements that often prevents us from reaching complete *Soul Health.* However, the wisdom we need to reach our unique radiance lies within our ability to access our inherent wisdom—our soul. In essence, it is our deepest ally; it inspires our path to true health. Only when we access this inherent wisdom—an entity unique to each of us—will we be able to create the landscape for our greatest sense of vitality. In other words, it is only when we align with our soul that we reach this much desired level of radiance.

The Soul Health Model: Aligning with Spirit for Radiant Living is your soul's practical guide to reaching your radiant vitality. In this book you will find a user-friendly metaphor for life-long wellness and optimal health. I invite you to grab a pen or highlighter as you read this book, so that you can identify key areas of your own life that need a bit of work. The chapters will take you through various exercises and activities designed both to assess your own branches of health, and also access your deepest ally.

Part One, **Exploring Soul Health,** explains the Soul Health Model in detail and not only provides a thorough understanding of ten essential elements of human health that must be balanced for optimal vitality, but also shows you how your soul influences and inspires each and every element within the branches of the human condition. The inter-relatedness of all the branches is explained to illustrate that if even one branch is unbalanced, it will have a significant impact on your overall vitality. Each element of your vitality will be explored through individual chapters, and brief assessments are included within each so you can learn more about that particular element in your life.

Part Two, Soul-Based Living, provides an extended Soul Health Assessment to help you fully understand your level of radiant vitality within each element at the deepest level—through your soul. This section also provides a Soul Health Plan and other exercises to guide you in creating your own optimal health as well as offer tips and suggestions for maintaining your new level of radiance once you reach it. The section especially emphasizes the idea of "soul stewardship" as a means to developing and maintaining a lifelong relationship with your inner ally—your soul.

Before you read further, here are a few things to keep in mind as you embark on your quest toward radiant health:

1. Know that like everything else in the human condition, soul health is a process. Just as your physical health requires ongoing attention, so does your soul's radiant health. You can think of this process as a sort of soul hygiene, which encourages awareness of your current state of overall health. Identification of areas that need some work or change will

help you invest in creating new habits and in an overall appreciation of yourself and your soul in the process.

2. There is no such thing as perfection. So, if you feel you must be perfect to reach soul health, rest easy. Even if you have a chronic physical or mental health issue, you can still work toward an enhanced state of radiant health. In fact, in doing so, you will very likely experience relief in those conditions. This is the point: Once you learn that radiant health is an interactive process concerning all aspects of your life, you will likely become more aware of what has contributed to your lack of radiant health as well as experience some relief as a result of this new awareness and any related changes you choose to make. In other words, instead of focusing on your *lack of* something, soul health is all about enhancing your life until you see what you really need—your soul—which has been there all along.

3. Soul health requires conscious choice. Like any other aspect of health, soul health only improves if you choose to do something to make it happen. If your dentist tells you to floss, you find a way to instill this habit into your daily life. Soul health requires the same—a conscious choice and some sort of action to accomplish it. In most cases, these actions are very simple, in others a bit more complex. But in either case, the conscious choice for change—your soul's evolution— is in your hands.

4. The pursuit of soul health is an evolutionary process. As you make even small changes toward your radiant health, you will experience ripples of improvements in many areas of your life. And each ripple will likely incite you to create more. If there is any hazard to pursuing soul health, it is that once

you realize how much better you can feel, and how many aspects of your life start to feel more vibrant, you really never want to stop improving your soul's radiance. The process of actualizing your soul, or allowing it to ascend, feels naturally satisfying—it leaves you wanting more and more. And if you invest in yourself, your ability to evolve is infinite—not to mention fun.

Soul health is a deeply personal process and journey—one which takes time and investment. But when we align with our deepest and wisest ally, the path to our radiant living appears right in front of us. We all deserve to reach our radiant vitality. And our soul knows just how to get us there.

Part One

Exploring Soul Health

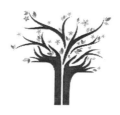

*Your work is to discover your world
and then with all your heart
give yourself to it.*
~~ Buddha

CHAPTER 1

THE SOUL HEALTH MODEL:
HOW SPIRIT INSPIRES WELL-BEING

The reason why the universe is eternal is that it does not live for itself, it gives life to others as it transforms. ~~ Lao Tzu

To say that our soul inspires us is like saying the sun is bright. It is so obvious that it is seldom voiced even by those who acknowledge its existence. In times of darkness, though, it is often difficult to remember that our soul is the generator of our very existence. When the human condition is out of balance—through stress, grief, or any other form of upheaval— it is extraordinarily difficult not to stay mired in our human condition. At times, it is nearly impossible to acknowledge that anything other than our pain could even exist.

The words "inspiration" and "inspire" evolved from the words "in spirit". So it only makes sense that our spirituality—our connection with our soul—is an inspiration to everyday life. When we are living fully "in spirit" we are more aligned with our soul than with the struggles of our human condition. But with the everyday challenges of our lives, it is often difficult to feel connected to, let alone inspired by, our soul as we decide what to do in any given situation or moment.

We have all had times when things seem to be going well and yet we still feel that something is missing. Try as we might, we cannot determine what that is. These are the times when our soul is trying to get our attention, but we are either misinterpreting or ignoring its call. The following chapters will explain that every emotion, physical symptom and other sign of *dis*-ease is simply a message to us—an inspiration from our soul—to rebalance our lives.

But what happens when so much is out of balance that we cannot even hear the inspiration, let alone decipher it? It is at these times that our overall well-being is the most threatened. When our well-being is fragile or vulnerable, our souls are at their lowest potential for evolution. However, when we tune in to the warning signs of imbalance that is when our souls are most likely to grow.

SOUL HEALTH

All the evolution we know of proceeds from the vague to the definite. ~~ Charles Sanders Peirce

Numerous studies illustrate the importance of spiritual and religious beliefs in recovering from various health problems. But little is written concerning how our soul interacts with—or inspires—our well-being to create overall wholeness. Even less is written about our soul's most natural state—its *evolution*.

In working with thousands of clients and workshop attendees, I have come to believe that there is a complex interplay between our overall well-being and the inspiration of our soul. This interplay represents the interaction between our ways of dealing with the human condition (the everyday struggles we encounter and our reactions to them) and our deepest and wisest core. Without an understanding of this complex interplay, not only do our human lives remain unbalanced, but our souls simply cannot fully evolve.

Unlike general wellness models, the Soul Health Model emphasizes the complex and key interplay between our human condition and our soul, not just a basic approach to life balance. Because our soul's evolution is dependent on both our life balance and a conscious awareness of our soul's influence, it is the combination of these forces that is unique to this model.

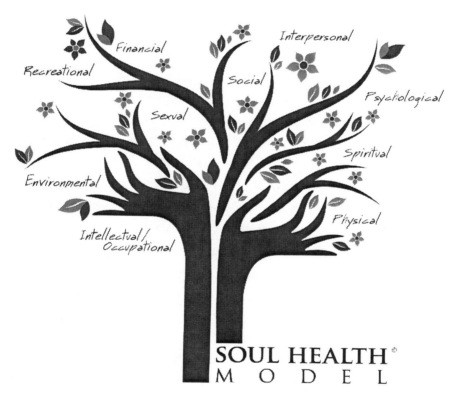

In the Soul Health Model, the soul is depicted as the life force within an ever-evolving tree. Much like the growth of an actual tree, which depends on sunlight, clean water and air, our soul's evolution depends on the health of the elements available to it and only thrives when the essentials of our existence are balanced and fulfilled. In the model, these elements represent the various aspects of our human condition—the health of our everyday life. Therefore, in order for an individual's soul to reach unimpeded growth, the individual must consciously maintain this healthy balance. This is not an easy feat given how persistently the issues of daily life get in the way. When we are overwhelmed, it is less and less likely that we will hear our soul. However, it is through physical, emotional, and other forms of *dis*-ease or lack of contentedness that our soul attempts to get our attention—to inspire us—in order to bring us back into balance and restore a sense of overall wholeness. Only then can our soul continue to evolve.

As depicted in the Soul Health Model the branches of the tree represent ten primary elements of the human condition. These branches must themselves be in balance, both separately and together for the soul to grow and evolve—and for us to flourish in our everyday lives. Each branch represents only one key to our overall sense of wholeness or soul health. These include Physical, Psychological, Social, Interpersonal, Social, Intellectual/Occupational, Financial, Environmental, Spiritual, Sexual, and Recreational (Fun & Leisure) branches of health. Each branch is but one bridge between the human condition and the soul. The entire tree represents the interplay between the two and illustrates the detrimental impact on our life when any one of the branches is not healthy. The model emphasizes that when one branch is "broken" it is impossible for the rest of the tree to remain unaffected. Even one unhealthy branch can have a traumatic impact on the soul's overall health.

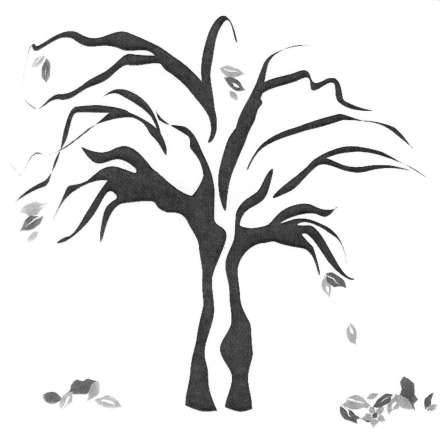

An injured or sick tree inherently knows what it needs in order to either heal or to sustain overall integrity until healing can take place. This is an automatic process—one that is programmed into the life force of a tree so that it will survive and even thrive beyond the impact of the injury. Unfortunately, we humans often lack this automatic response. We are less conscious of what we need than a tree is and often less active in rebalancing our lives. Because our lives are so much more complex than that of a tree, we often miss the cues for when one or more branches of our human condition are threatened and in need of healing. With respect to our overall soul health, we can suffer greatly if we remain unaware of the entirety of our daily needs as well as the complexity between the key aspects of our lives that impact our overall wholeness.

THE 10 BRANCHES OF HEALTH

As noted, each branch of health represents an aspect of the human condition that affects our overall well-being. Following are brief descriptions of all branches. Future chapters will describe each branch in greater detail, but for now, become acquainted with what is required for each element to be strong:

Physical: Freedom from physical disease or other signs of ill health. Important factors to maintain this branch include good nutrition, adequate sleep, basic physical fitness, reasonable mobility, adequate energy and motivation. Although the physical branch is often most acknowledged, the nine branches that follow are essential to optimal well-being.

Psychological: Freedom from emotional *dis*-ease and the ability to maintain a sense of contentment. This branch emphasizes an overall sense of well-being, self-esteem, positive self-image, and of course emotional health—including freedom from depression, anxiety, or other psychological disturbances. This branch also accounts for our *perception* of the rest of the tree and how balanced our lives are.

Social: This branch represents the people—and animals—that we value in our lives. These include family, friends, partners, pets, neighbors, co-workers, clergy, and any others with whom we have contact. Introverts and extroverts may need very different numbers and even kinds of relationships, but what matters is having important contacts to create connectedness or community.

Interpersonal: I separate this branch from the Social branch primarily to stress the idea of *quality* in relationships. This branch reflects healthy boundaries, good communication, a good balance of independence an inter-dependence with others (good give and take relationships), mutual respect and equality within one's relationships. People can have many social contacts in their lives, but if the dynamics of these relationships are not healthy, they will have an enormously detrimental impact on their overall well-being.

Intellectual/Occupational: In general, this branch emphasizes the need for mental stimulation regardless of gainful employment. Without intellectual challenge and genuine interest, people become bored. It is important that life provides engaging in daily tasks, curiosity about people and ideas, acquisition of new knowledge, and a general quest for learning. Regardless of a person's employment status, intellectual health is essential to overall well-being.

Environmental: Environmental wellness depends on clean, safe, healthy and generally satisfying surroundings. To sustain this branch requires climate, good air quality, sound control, lack of clutter and some degree of control over other external factors that might undermine environmental health and well-being. These might also include aspects of the "emotional environment" such as ongoing corporate stress, family tension, and threats to personal safety.

Financial: To be healthy, this branch depends on having ample financial resources to meet our basic needs. Spending within our limits, preventing major debt, saving for the future, investing well, planning for retirement and developing healthy ideas about the use of money are all ways we can maintain the health of this branch. Particularly in times of financial crisis, this branch can have a tremendous impact on every other branch of health. Our beliefs about wealth and abundance also come into play with this branch of health.

Spiritual: Although this model provides an abstract representation of the interaction between our human condition and our soul, it takes active and deliberate attention to our spiritual life for our soul to evolve. This branch depends on a healthy sense of inner peace and/or a belief in higher power. Having a healthy spiritual branch doesn't necessarily include the practice of religion. However, it does include regular participation in "centering" techniques such as prayer, meditation, and ritual, as well as an unconditional and nonjudgmental mindset toward the world.

Sexual: Because societal and personal issues so greatly affect our attitudes about our sexuality, this branch plays a key role in overall well-being. This branch includes healthy sexual boundaries and an understanding of appropriate sexual activity with self and others. Because so many people—women in particular—have experienced sexual trauma, it is important that any such experiences are fully explored and resolved in order for the soul to be unimpeded in its search for peace and ultimate growth. This branch also depends on a person's ability to see sexual activity as an intimate act of relationship, not simply a way to fill basic, individual needs.

Recreation (Fun & Leisure): This branch may seem more like a luxury than a necessity for overall well-being, but I have found it to be an essential and too often overlooked part of life. Leisure activities— attending sports events, theater performances and art exhibits, exercising, reading, writing, painting, playing games, cooking, vacationing, watching television and movies and so on —help us to relax and decompress from everyday stress. Anything that invokes appropriate laughter and lightheartedness, as well as both physical and emotional release of tension acts as good medicine. Although our society seems to underestimate the value of fun and leisure to our overall health, a person just has to look at the overall tree to recognize how this branch can alleviate the stressors of the human condition when other branches are unbalanced.

The branches of the tree are so interconnected that if one is damaged or out of balance, the rest are directly affected—there is no escaping this. For instance, the financial stress of someone who has been laid off during a bad economy will eventually weaken all the branches of the tree. The individual will immediately experience stress (*psychological*), which in turn can create health problems (*physical*), cause them to isolate from friendly activities (*social*) to conserve money (*financial*), cause marital conflict or disagreement with friends (*interpersonal*), lower a person's libido (*sexual*), affect the person's faith or belief system about life events (*spiritual*), and so on. As you can see, it is impossible for the entirety of the tree—the human condition— to remain strong when even one branch is damaged.

OUR SOUL'S HEALTH AND EVOLUTION

In the illustration of the Soul Health Model, the trunk of the tree houses the soul and is depicted by hands reaching upward toward our most natural state—our soul's expansive evolution. Only when the branches of the tree—our human condition—are in full balance can our soul truly blossom. So, when we experience discomfort about events or situations in our lives, it is our soul's way of getting our attention and informing us that something is amiss—something is darkening our view and keeping us from fully blooming. Our discomfort is our soul's way of inspiring us to change—to adjust something within one or more branches or even to prune away what no longer fits. An actual tree doesn't need something to inspire it to change. It just knows there is mending to be done to a broken limb or malnourished trunk. However, humans must learn to view discontent or unhappiness as the cue to assess and balance the key elements of their lives in order to maintain the equilibrium between human condition and our soul. It is when the soul's growth is impeded that we feel emotional or physical discomfort, and this leaves us feeling far away from our inherent desire to thrive.

Our soul inherently knows what we need in order to thrive, but we often get mired in our everyday life—our human condition—to the point where we ignore the vital cues that are right before us. We have been conditioned to think and feel a certain way by those around us and this is often to the detriment of our wholeness—which directly reflects the necessities of our soul. Understanding the interplay between our overall health or wholeness and our inner voice—or inspiration—of our soul is what can bring our fullest and richest experience of what it means to be human. This also creates a deep awareness about how much richer life can be than we have been taught to expect. If we are meant to evolve, we must balance the ten key aspects of our human condition with the inner voice of our soul to find our most radiant balance of health.

REDESIGNING OUR SOUL'S LANDSCAPE

Anyone who tends to house plants or a garden knows that the two key tricks to keeping plants alive are 1) to clean out the dead or wilting leaves, stems, or branches and 2) to provide water and nourishment to promote growth. These concepts are pretty simple. Unfortunately, our quest for radiant health is often not as simple.

When I use the Soul Health Model with clients, it helps them clean out parts of their lives that aren't working and to fill up, or enhance, their lives by using the inspiration of their soul as a guide. It may seem that finding and listening to the voice of our soul is the more challenging of these tasks in our own evolution. Many books have been written to help people identify this inner voice. However, in my work as a therapist, it is clearly the cleaning out of unhealthy aspects of the human condition that is the most challenging part of our growth because we may become attached to certain people, habits, and objects despite how unhealthy they may be for us.

Any attempt to hear the voice of your soul from an untended or cluttered human "garden" can muffle its true voice and/or lead you to misinterpret the message. However, in actively cleaning out emotional, psychological, social and other debris, you become able to decipher the message of your soul more clearly. The ultimate goal is to learn to utilize the voice of your soul in the process of balancing the ten essential aspects—or branches—within your life. In this way, you learn to work in tandem with your soul to create a new and more fulfilling landscape for your life—you create your conscious evolution.

BRIEF SOUL ASSESSMENT

Although a full assessment will be offered in Part Two, please take a moment to complete the following Brief Soul Assessment. Later in the book, as each chapter unfolds, you will be asked to complete more in-depth assessments of your soul health, but reading the rest of the chapters in Part One will help you to fully understand each branch represented in the questionnaire.

Brief Soul Survey

Please circle the number that applies best.
O represents "not at all healthy" and 10 represents "completely healthy"

Overall Sense of Health
Not at all 0 1 2 3 4 5 6 7 8 9 10 Completely

Physical Health
(fitness/exercise, nutrition, lack of disease/illness)

Not at all 0 1 2 3 4 5 6 7 8 9 10 Completely

Psychological Health
(emotions, thoughts, self-esteem, lack of *dis*-ease)

Not at all 0 1 2 3 4 5 6 7 8 9 10 Completely

Social Health
(friends, family, colleagues, social support, pets)
Not at all 0 1 2 3 4 5 6 7 8 9 10 Completely

Interpersonal Health
(personal/family dynamics, communication, boundaries, respect)

Not at all 0 1 2 3 4 5 6 7 8 9 10 Completely

Intellectual/Occupational Health
(mental stimulation, occupational fulfillment, curiosity)

Not at all 0 1 2 3 4 5 6 7 8 9 10 Completely
Environmental Health
(housing, safety, climate, clutter, sustainability)

Not at all 0 1 2 3 4 5 6 7 8 9 10 Completely

Financial Health
(wealth/debt management, planning for future, spending habits)

Not at all 0 1 2 3 4 5 6 7 8 9 10 Completely

Spiritual Health
(inner peace, meaning/purpose, belief in higher power)

Not at all 0 1 2 3 4 5 6 7 8 9 10 Completely

Sexual Health
(intimacy, passion, safety, satisfaction)

Not at all 0 1 2 3 4 5 6 7 8 9 10 Completely

Recreational Health (Fun and Leisure)
(leisure, entertainment, relaxation, fun)

Not at all 0 1 2 3 4 5 6 7 8 9 10 Completely

In completing the Brief Soul Assessment, it is not uncommon for individuals to rate themselves higher in overall health, and then re-evaluate rating their health on each specific branch. This is simply because we tend not to be aware of the interconnectedness of all the branches until we spend some time thinking about them. For now, just use this information to remain conscious of areas that you feel need work along the way.

When you do a full assessment of every branch of your soul health, you will become aware that some sections need some pruning, while others need to be fortified for more growth and greater fullness of the tree. Also, if your tree doesn't feel firmly rooted, it might be that some foundational work needs to be done in order for you to know your soul and your values better. Or perhaps you lack a feeling of being grounded or balanced in your life overall. This usually means that either your "soul sense"—a grasp of who you are and what your values are—needs work or that you have too much going on in life and aren't fully anchored to your own priorities. Deep down, we generally know when something is not quite right; we just don't know how to access whatever it is and how to fix our own personal tree of life. The Soul Health Model will help you identify and prioritize what needs attention.

TO HEAL OR TO EVOLVE—THAT IS THE QUESTION!

Current literature offers many options for healing from both physical and emotional problems. The point is to reduce or eliminate the impact of any physical symptoms or emotional discontent. However, to me, healing is only a part of the story. The mind-body-spirit approach does not separate any of these key elements of health from the others. The Soul Health Model emphasizes an inseparable connection that extends beyond physical, emotional, and other concerns and relates to the health of the soul as well. In other words, it redefines health to include, and rely upon, a conscious understanding of the intricate relationship between health or well-being and the undeniable influence of our soul.

The ongoing challenge with modern medicine is that practitioners generally only have time to screen for one or two aspects of overall health—*if* we are lucky. If medical providers don't assess all branches of health, they miss critical information about the whole person, let alone the health of the soul. They can easily overlook key information not only about the kind of healing that's needed, but also about measures that might help patients evolve *beyond* their current level of vitality—or lack thereof. Given that most practitioners will not have studied the soul's power to advance health and healing, patients who wish to tap into that power will need a firm grasp of ten key aspects of human health and an ability to recognize and act upon the intuitions and inner knowing that comes from the soul.

The following chapters will explore the ten branches of health in much more detail. As your knowledge of these key aspects of human health unfolds, you will also gain a fuller understanding of how soul health promotes the evolution of your soul.

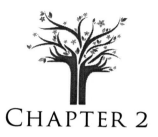

CHAPTER 2

SOUL SURVIVAL:
TOOLS FOR CONSCIOUS EVOLUTION

*I believe that man will not merely endure. He will prevail.
He is immortal, not because he alone among creatures has
an inexhaustible voice, but because he has a soul, a spirit
capable of compassion and sacrifice and endurance.* ~~
taken from William Faulkner's Nobel Prize Speech

The survival of our species depends not only on our ability to maintain and improve physical health but also the health of our souls. For years scientists have stated that the human body has, for the most part, evolved as far as it is going to. Therefore, we must turn our focus to the vitality of our soul if we are not only to survive, but to thrive, which will allow us to evolve beyond our current state of being.

Ancient civilizations and native cultures were, and still are, much more in tune with an inner essence,—one that is not only concerned with themselves but is interwoven with everything else— other individuals, their society as a group, their surroundings, the

Earth, all of its elements and species, and all other aspects that fuel their existence—the sun, the moon, the trees, the wind, the rain, the food on their table and in their fields, the clothes on their backs, the stones under their feet, and each speck of dust on the ground. Such civilizations need very little from our modern world in order to survive. They live much more simply, yet "wholly" with less complaint about what they don't have and more appreciation for what they do. However, each new generation of industrialized, high technology cultures seems to put the soul further and further out of mind or out of reach. Modern societies have lost track, not only of any connection with the Earth and with each other, but, more dangerously, with our own most vital center—our own soul.

The word soul has, in some ways, been so loosely and carelessly used that it has lost its meaning. Few could aptly define it, let alone gain access to it. In our feeble attempts to reconnect with our souls, we have named anything from automobiles to arena football teams after it, created resort and spa names that promise to nurture it, released a multitude of articles, books, audiotapes and videos professing the importance of it, and to date produced nearly 1.2 billion Google hits related to it. Is this a step in the right direction? Maybe. Maybe not.

There is much more to reconnecting with the soul than simply acknowledging it is there or romanticizing what it is. Learning how to work with our soul in the course of daily life is no longer a simple option, it is the only way to truly evolve beyond the human condition. Few people consciously engage in their physical and psychological health let alone in the question of their role in the progression of the human species. Our world would not be in such frightening disarray if we were all firmly grounded in our soul and working consciously toward our own and our species' overall growth and awareness. There would be no war, no destruction, no discrimination, no preventable illnesses, no major debt, no political uprising, no volatile stock markets, no hunger, no homelessness—not much of anything that afflicts our world today. There would be no need for any of this. If every person actively worked on the health and evolution of his or her soul, there is little doubt that the world would be a far better place.

Suffice it to say that the word soul in this book refers to our innermost essence or sense of knowing. It is the nucleus of all that we are—the core of our existence. It is the pinpoint of light within us that tells us something is right or wrong, whether we listen to that message or not. It is the gut instinct that tells us whether we are doing something that is helpful or damaging to our own or another's well-being, whether or not we choose to act accordingly. It is also the tie that binds us to each and every other soul--- one that creates our universal community. Simply put, the soul is the key not only to our survival, but to our evolution as well. To know your soul is to know true health—regardless of the state of the body alone. As Ray Charles said, "What is a soul? It's like electricity—we don't really know what it is, but it's a force that can light a room!"

THE ROLE OF CONSCIOUSNESS

Nothing can cure the soul but the senses, just as nothing can cure the senses but the soul. ~~ Oscar Wilde.

How does one evolve? By consciously choosing to do so. If the human body has evolved about as far as it is going to, then we must rely on our minds and our souls together—a conscious *knowing* of how to create a radiant life. Intellect alone just won't suffice.

Although humans have more advanced intellect than all other species, we often lag behind when it comes to conscious living. Many other species are far more conscious—that is alert, attentive, and focused than we tend to be. They are also more trusting of their innermost awareness and instinct. Take, for instance, animals who sense danger—a storm, earthquake, hurricane, tsunami, or tornado—long before it is anywhere near the vicinity in which they live. These animals are attuned to their inner knowing or alert system, and they adjust their patterns accordingly, for the sake of their survival. They follow their consciousness about impending danger without the use of advanced intellect. They not only hear, but also heed their inner awareness.

However, with the evolution of the human intellect has come a dimming of our inner knowledge—a dismissal of our soul. Our quest for cognitive intelligence has disconnected us from our most vital ally. What would be possible if we reconnected our mind with our soul? What would happen if we plugged back into this vital source and actually listened to it? What sort of synthesis of awareness would occur if we used both intellect and our soul to guide our life?

The term consciousness means to be "in a state of being aware especially of something within oneself." If we rely on our intellect alone we will inevitably miss the vital information we need in order to evolve. This is where *radical consciousness* comes in—a term I use to describe our path to evolution. To be radical means "to have something arise from or going to a root or source." Therefore, to be radically conscious means "to go straight to the meaning of something within." In the case of health, if we rely solely on our own or others' *intellect*, we very likely overlook what we really need in order to feel optimally vibrant or healthy. We take information from the outside and apply it—often blindly, without ever assessing whether it feels right as we follow this external advice. The outcome may appear to have short-term positive effects, but only as long as we can sustain them.

For example, there are thousands of weight-loss strategies available which can produce significant, but temporary results. Many are designed for short-term effects that are not sustainable for the duration of our lives. Rarely does a diet plan discuss the need to listen within to determine what your body needs at any given time. The truth is our bodies need different things at different times, and different people often need different levels or types of nutrients to feel healthy and satisfied. No diet plan can predict what an individual needs with 100 percent accuracy; none will meet the needs of your body at every given moment. The body shifts from moment to moment, day to day, season to season, year to year, decade to decade. However, if we don't follow these prescribed diet plans to a T, then we are left to feel like failures and start the cycle of weight gain and temporary weight loss all over again.

Most animals in the wild eat when they are hungry and drink when they are thirsty. If they stop eating, it means they are either full or sick. For them, it is simple. They listen within to determine whether they search for food or take a nap. Yes, they have much more simple needs, but they also assess *and* tend to them more effectively than most people. They sense what they need and then they act accordingly.

For humans, conscious living is more complex. It takes a certain amount of work for us to reach this state because our needs are more complicated—psychological, social, interpersonal, intellectual, interpersonal, spiritual and so on. For us, conscious living requires a deep awareness of how the body, mind, and soul function together to create "whole" health—a sense that all aspects of our life feel balanced or complete. By choosing to live more consciously we can more effectively and directly assess our innermost needs—our soul wisdom—to achieve a more radiant human experience. We all have hunches about life,—many of which we don't follow. Our intellect, or rational thinking, has overpowered our inner knowing to the point where we take many detours regardless of what our instincts tell us. We have lost the art of living and replaced it with the science instead by acting primarily on what our thoughts tell us rather than how our soul may instruct us to proceed. In doing so we have made our lives increasingly empty and unhealthy, always seeming to look outside ourselves for what we sense is missing. This is clearly the wrong direction, for otherwise more people would feel fulfilled and content. Therefore, becoming radically conscious is essential not only to our experience of radiant health, but also to our evolution of mind and soul together.

KNOWING SOUL

The soul is so far from being a monad that we have not only to interpret other souls to our self but to interpret our self to our self. ~~ T. S. Eliot

To know true health is to know your soul, and no one else can know your soul like you do. No one can interpret it from the outside. Sadly, too few people do know their souls, let alone listen to them. Most ignore inner stirrings and messages live their lives the modern world seems to dictate. We trust the outside world more than the one within. This is not to say we shouldn't follow certain social mores and responsibilities, just that we are rarely taught to seek our inner wisdom. We are instructed to use our brains but not to develop the ability to hear an inner voice.

And so we remain discontent. Our uneasiness arises from doing certain things that don't *feel* right to us and perhaps ignoring other things that might feel right but that we are conditioned to avoid. Our brains may tell us to do, or not do, something, but our souls say something otherwise. This is how we experience regret— by lamenting what we did or failed to do in the past while deeply *wondering* how life might have turned out differently. We may know something is missing but we don't know what "it" is. We *sense* a void of some sort even if we can't identify the source.

To know your soul is to develop an intense and deep relationship with it—to regard it as your most vital ally. This requires a faithful trust in yourself and the inner workings of your evolving self. The volume of your inner voice needs to be turned up and the volume on your intellect turned down so you are able to hear both, but with a keen focus on what your soul is communicating. Sometimes your soul will instruct you to do something that seems illogical to your mind, but is actually more aligned with what you need in order to reach radiant health. This "soul intelligence" will guide you much more directly toward optimal health and overall satisfaction in life more quickly than the advice of others. Your "soul IQ" will provide all the answers you need, simply by helping you to hear and trust the messages from within.

I have taught in various medical and healthcare institutions, and the main emphasis was always on the doctor-patient relationship—how to make the patient feel heard, even during a five minute appointment. However, no one talks to patients about listening to their soul for the benefit of their health. No one sits them down to explain the ten key aspects of human life and asks, "What do you need in order to feel 'whole' in each one of these?" The medical profession doesn't focus on what it takes to make people feel fully vibrant and radiant in their overall health

Soul health is not only about balancing the aspects of everyday life in order to feel whole, it is also about reconnecting with our innermost ally in such a way that we never lose vitality again. It is about combining intellectual awareness about what is good in the everyday world with clear choices offered by the wisdom of our soul. Soul health is also about creating a strong relationship with yourself that makes it possible to commit to your growth and evolution as a soul-based being. This allows not only a deeper understanding of what we need as individuals, but also an expansive awareness of the true radiant vitality of our soul.

Committing to soul health not only makes it possible to create a radiant life regardless of whatever ails us, it also lets us evolve beyond some of these ailments. It makes it possible to capture and embrace our radiance and *decide* to make the very most of our precious and irreplaceable life.

WHERE DOES THE SOUL GO FROM HERE?

This book is used most effectively when you allow your soul to answer the questions and explore its needs with help but not interference from intellect. Here are a few quick exercises that will help you access your soul wisdom rather than relying on your thoughts alone. The three quickest ways to know if your soul is answering are these:

1. If there is any emotion involved (whether fear or excitement!), then the answer is not soul-based. There is no emotion in our soul response—emotion is only an aspect of the human condition. The soul itself does not need emotion in order to guide us, although we might experience a human emotion as we receive soul-based guidance. The soul provides the what *is*, not the what *ifs,* which are always a product of our thoughts. Therefore, if the answer arises as a result of an emotion, it is brain-based; however, if the emotion arises as a *response* to the answer, then it is soul-based. In other words, sometimes we don't want to admit what the answer is because of the emotion attached to it, but it the answer is our truth nevertheless.

2. If your response feels like a gut reaction rather than a worrisome thought, it is soul-based. If you find yourself thinking too much or scanning your brain for the answer, you are searching in the wrong place. Our truth resides in our gut—or our solar plexus area, which is located slightly below our rib cage and above our navel. It is where we experience the sucker punches of life, when we know something doesn't

feel right, or when we have left something undone. It is the house of regret. It is also the house of peace when an answer does feel right. There is a comfort or contentment when we feel we are moving in the right direction or making a decision that works for us. Our gut reactions tell us we have found our inner wisdom— the inner sanctum of our soul. So, if you have a gut response to a question, it is a soul-based awareness or answer.

3. If it takes more than a few seconds to answer for you to receive an answer, it is not soul-based. Soul-based responses are generally instantaneous. They arise very quickly and with much clarity. This is why they are gut reactions—they come directly out of your inner wisdom and require no deliberation. The answer is just what it is. And with each soul-based answer comes a self-induced affirmation—an inner sense or connection with the soul. You just *know* it's the right answer, regardless of any action it might require. Note that on some occasions your gut or soul may not have an answer—and this is simply a sign that it is not yet time for you to know what you are asking. Be patient. The answer will come when it is supposed to.

As you proceed through the following chapters, which relate to the ten branches of health, consider using the strategies below to explore and assess your needs for each branch. These can be used for both the "cleaning out" and the "filling up" process for each branch.

EXERCISE ONE—THE YES-NO ANSWER

Ask yourself yes-no questions. For instance, in the physical branch—if you ask yourself, "Do I need to exercise more?" you will likely get a very quick yes or no. This question gets right to the gut of the answer—right to the soul—, and can be used each step of the way.

EXERCISE TWO—THE GUT QUESTION

If the yes-no question doesn't apply or doesn't seem to be giving you a response, ask yourself, "What does my gut tell me I need (or don't need)?" This will direct your answer away from your brain and open you to receiving the wisdom of your soul—your gut reaction or response. For example, if you are assessing the social branch and there is a friendship or relationship you are struggling with, ask something like "What does my gut tell me to do about this person?" You may not like the answer that arises, but it is certain to be the right one for your soul's health.

EXERCISE THREE—AUTOMATIC WRITING

Automatic writing is a technique used to spontaneously explore the possibilities and probabilities of a given question or concern. The object is to uncover your unconscious wisdom about the question to make the answer more conscious. You simply sit down with some blank paper, write down a question at the top of the paper, then allow your thoughts to stream freely as you write down the responses. There is really no thinking involved—you simply document whatever stream of words or thoughts arise without having to problem-solve a single thing. For example, in assessing the spiritual branch of health you could write down the question "What do I need to feel more spiritual?" Then allow yourself simply to jot down the responses that arise.

Keep in mind that finding and creating soul health is a process, one we must periodically reassess and adjust in order to meet our ever-changing needs. It is a very conscious process, one that requires a commitment to our self and to our soul in order to reach our radiant vitality. As you proceed through the following chapters, try not to become bogged down in all of the things you want to change or improve upon in your life. The idea of soul health is not to overwhelm, but rather to enhance the radiance available to you. In doing so, see the bright light of your soul as never before. Only your soul can provide the wisdom to reach your true vitality.

Chapter 3

Physical Health:
From Basic Needs to Body Language

You don't have a soul. You are a soul. You have a body. ~~ C.S. Lewis

Health is a deeply personal thing. From the common cold to chronic illness, every physical ailment has an impact on how we experience the human condition. Any indication that we are not well threatens the quality or duration of our existence, and, more seriously, it affects the core of our being—our soul. Our health is multidimensional; it involves each and every aspect of our lives, which, cannot help but suffer along with the body. When we are ill, we often feel down emotionally. Our relationships suffer, and in some cases we lose them. Our jobs may be jeopardized, we neglect our surroundings, struggle to find or maintain inner peace (which may go out the window altogether), lose sexual interest, perhaps lose money as well, and certainly are not in the right frame of mind for good fun and leisure.

In 1955, Pierre Teilhard de Chardin, a French Jesuit priest and philosopher, wrote in *Le Phénomène Humain* (The Human

Phenomenon) that "We are not human beings having a spiritual experience. We are spiritual beings having a human experience." And there is nothing more human than our physical bodies. They may be finished evolving, but they are necessary to the soul's continued evolution.

People spend an inordinate amount of money each year not only on health and physical fitness products, but on beauty products as well, which demonstrates the value they place on the state and appearance of their bodies. However, this focus on the physical body often ignores other aspects of overall well-being. This chapter explains the complex effects that our physical health can have on all branches of our vitality and illustrates how our body's health reflects the health of our soul.

THE SOUL CONNECTION

The human body is the best picture of human soul. ~~ Ludwig Wittgenstein

Theories about the mind-body connection have dated back to about 430 BCE when Hippocrates attempted to explain the intricate and surprising connections between mental phenomena and physiological order. Later, Plato advocated for physical exercise as a way to develop the mind, with his ideal being the harmonious perfection of body, mind, and psyche. However, it really wasn't until 1937, when Joseph Pilates wrote about the balance of the mind and body in *Your Health,* that the modern wellness movement got underway. This was the first time that such a balance was suggested as a means to prevent physical illness through the balance of other aspects of life. Yet it still took until 1976 for the National Wellness Institute (NWI) to unveil their model of health, which included in overall physical and psychological wellness, four other components— social, environmental, spiritual and intellectual.

As noted in the introduction to this book, it took until a few years ago for the Soul Health Model to evolve as well. I used the NWI's model for over a decade before I, too, found missing links (the sexual, financial, interpersonal, and recreational aspects of health), the most critical of these aspects being the inherent influence of the soul on each and every other aspect of health. In essence, the soul is at the very core of our overall well-being. From a deeper level than we normally experience in daily life, our soul speaks out—often in ways our minds do not yet readily understand,— and influences our desires, preferences, behaviors, reactions, and responses to all other aspects of life. The result is what we generally regard as physical health, whatever its condition. When we begin deliberately to take our soul into our assessment of overall health, it adds a new and unmistakable dimension. It guides us to radiant health by instructing us for what we need not only to fulfill the physical branch of health, but all others as well.

The human body is a barometer of all other aspects of health—psychological, social, spiritual and so on. It indicates that our lives are balanced or unbalanced, diseased or in a state of *dis*-ease, regardless of whether we make an attempt to rectify the other branches. Cicero said "Diseases of the soul are more dangerous and more numerous than those of the body"; however, our soul's house—the human body—is the primary gauge for our soul's afflictions. When we are stressed or distressed we develop physical symptoms that coincide. When we are lonely we say that our hearts ache. If the climate changes our bodies must adapt to remain comfortable. When our finances shrink, our waistlines may grow or dwindle depending on the situation. If our social supports fade, our visits to the doctor may increase. When we lose a job we sometimes gain an ulcer. If we lack inner peace, we often develop the physical symptoms of stress. No matter which branch of the tree of soul health is affected, it is often the body that reacts.

Henry David Thoreau made the connection between the soul and physical health: "Good for the body is the work of the body, good for the soul the work of the soul, and good for either the work of the other." It stands to reason, then, that in order to truly understand and embrace physical health one must also understand and embrace the influence of the soul.

THE PHYSICAL BRANCH OF HEALTH

Yet this is health: To have a body functioning so perfectly that when its few simple needs are met it never calls attention to its own existence. ~~ Bertha Stuart Dyment

Although the physical branch of health is the most basic, for many it is the most multidimensional as well, not only because of the intricacies of human anatomy, but also because it reflects every other branch of health.

What do you think of when you think about physical health? Most define a "good bill of health" as the lack of any illness, injury, or disease. However, this definition doesn't fully describe what it means to experience optimal health.

Ask yourself: On a scale of 1 to 10, 10 being perfect *physical health*—how would you rate yourself? What would it take to score a 10? What would you need to add to your life—or remove? How does it feel to think about making changes in order to reach your optimal health? What—or who—is getting in your way? How ready are you to experience optimal physical health? How ready are you to make any necessary changes?

Do you have an illness that has been diagnosed by a physician? When was it diagnosed? What was going on in the various branches your life around the time you first experienced symptoms? Do you take medication to relieve physical symptoms of something caused by stress? Are you addressing the stressor,—or just the related physical symptom?

In reading these questions, you might notice your mind trailing off to consider what other aspects of your life would have to change in order for you to experience full physical health. You might experience some distress or discomfort as you realize that in order to reach optimal physical health you will have to explore other facets of life as well. Precisely! Something might not be sitting right with you as you ponder your physical health.

These stirrings come from the soul. They are your soul's voice waking up to the possibility that you are actually listening to what it might take to reach physical health. They are your innermost ally's way of celebrating the potential for positive change. Although these stirrings might feel uncomfortable, it is only because they have been muffled and ignored for so long. This is not to say that by addressing the other aspects of health you are assured that a serious medical illness will disappear, but it is entirely possible that you will experience a new level of well-being—of radiance— despite the physical condition.

COMMON HEALTH FACTORS

Health is a big word. It embraces not the body only, but the mind and spirit as well;…and not today's pleasure and pain alone but the whole being and outlook of a man. ~~ James H. West

When you go to the doctor, the primary aspects of health that are discussed include evidence of a physical illness or disease, the balance of physical fitness and healthy nutrition, issues related to sleep, concerns about energy and possibly motivation, levels of mobility, and changes in overall health. However, a more comprehensive assessment of the physical branch of health is important in understanding the full context of soul health.

The following questionnaire may look much like what you have filled out in a physician's office. However, the difference lies in how you answer it. As you read through the questions, listen deeply within for the inner stirrings of your soul. It is the voice that is telling you 1) whether or not you are answering the question honestly, and 2) whether deep down you know that something is unbalanced regarding that particular aspect of your physical health. If you hesitate to answer a question, it is a sign that something needs work. Don't be alarmed; this awareness simply allows you to identify the elements of this branch that need either cleaning out or filling up.

QUESTIONNAIRE FOR THE PHYSICAL BRANCH OF HEALTH

On a scale of 1 to 10, rate the level of your health within each area described. A 10 describes optimal, radiant health, while a 1 describes an almost complete lack of health within the given aspect of the physical branch. Remember, this questionnaire is designed to create a roadmap to overall radiant health. It is not meant to overwhelm you.

Physical Fitness

1. ____ I am satisfied with the health of my physical body.
2. ____ I engage in regular physical activity, exercise, and stretching.
3. ____ I have full and comfortable mobility.
4. ____ I have enough energy and motivation.
5. ____ I am fully aware of what my body needs.
6. ____ My body is strong and vibrant.
7. ____ I maintain a healthy weight.

Nutrition

1. ____ I eat healthy and nutritious food daily.
2. ____ I understand food labels and use them to select what I eat.
3. ____ I eat a balanced diet with appropriate portion sizes.
4. ____ I know what vitamins and minerals my body needs and eat food that provides them.
5. ____ I drink enough water to feel fully hydrated.
6. ____ I eat when I'm hungry and stop when I'm full.

Sleep

1. ____ I get enough sleep to feel rested throughout the day.
2. ____ I sleep deeply and soundly.
3. ____ I follow a regular sleep schedule.
4. ____ I am able to sleep without the use of medication.

Illness

1. ____ I am free of physical illness.
2. ____ I follow what my healthcare provider recommends to care for my physical health.
3. ____ I am proactive in preventing illness (self-exams, regular exercise, healthy nutrition, etc.).
4. ____ I do not have frequent minor illnesses (headaches, colds, infections, injuries).
5. ____ I take a proactive approach toward returning to health when I am ill.

Healthy Habits

1. ____ I use no tobacco products.
2. ____ I drink two or fewer alcoholic beverages per week.
3. ____ I limit my caffeine intake to the equivalent of two six-ounce cups of coffee per day.
4. ____ I practice physical safety, using protective equipment such as gloves or goggles when necessary.
5. ____ I use sunscreen regularly.
6. ____ I do self-exams as recommended (breasts, testicles, skin, etc.).
7. ____ I brush and floss my teeth as recommended.
8. ____ I see all of my healthcare providers as recommended.
9. ____ I drive safely.
10. ____ I practice safe sex.
11. ____ I use non-toxic cleaning and other household products.

While taking the questionnaire, your internal barometer—your soul—was influencing how you answered. You likely had a gut reaction to each question, whether you liked the answer that came with it or not. This is your truth—your inner wisdom speaking on behalf of your overall radiant health. For instance, in answering whether you maintain a healthy weight, your gut may have answered no—since nearly 66 percent of people in America are overweight. Intellectually, we understand what a healthy weight is. However, the responsive stirring you feel within is your soul's desire to reach or return to a healthy physical weight. Your body *knows* that it doesn't feel good being overweight, and, your soul reminds you of this by creating a sense of discomfort—a longing to balance your life in order to experience optimal health. In this way, your soul is telling you to get on the ball to feel better!

In fact, in our culture, it is likely that weight is the primary barometer of our soul health. I have worked with hundreds of people who are overweight and/or dealing with one eating disorder or another. Those with problem eating are clearly not at peace with themselves or their lives. And since our bodies are the barometers of our soul, it is not hard to recognize that many people are not experiencing radiant soul health when it comes to weight. The trick is to identify the branch or branches of overall soul health that are creating the problem. If you believe this is as easy as eating less and moving more, you are wrong. And your soul will confirm this.

Another example is your answer to the question about personal safety. Your answer may have reflected a low incidence of using these protectors, while your soul is reminding you of the times you didn't. This holds true for everything from the time you got sunburned because you didn't use sunscreen to the day when your dentist said you had a cavity and knew all too well you hadn't been taking care of your teeth.

Fitness and nutrition are obvious factors in your physical health.

However, they are also essential to your soul health and evolution. When we don't attend to the needs of the body, we are neglecting the soul as well. Research repeatedly demonstrates the positive benefits of physical activity on every system within the body—cardio, pulmonary, endocrine, limbic, immune, and so on. Increasing research on nutrition also illustrates the importance of conscious eating in order to nourish the body for optimal health as well as for the deterrence of preventable diseases.

Regarding sleep, no one feels good when deprived of it. Our mood changes, our health habits change, and over time we start to see physical effects as well. New research links sleep problems with obesity, heart disease, high blood pressure, low immune function, and other physical conditions. No one suffering from chronic sleep issues feels close to their soul.

When our body feels good, we feel good. When it doesn't, our soul suffers, not only because physically we are not up to par, but also because as a result of suboptimal functioning, we are less able to attend to other needs as well—particularly those of our soul.

Thus our soul needs our body to remain well. It is the only way it can survive, thrive, and evolve. Thoreau confirmed this when he said "... good for either, the work of the other." It is important to remember that our body is truly the barometer of our soul, and if we learn to interpret the messages from within, we can often rebalance our lives for the benefit of our overall health.

However, what about all of the healthy behaviors we avoid? Why don't we exercise more? Why don't we choose to eat healthy foods? Why don't we go to the doctor, take our vitamins, or take better care of our bodies overall? Despite their inner stirrings, many overlook or deliberately avoid the messages from their soul that are sent through their physical body.

Body "Language"

Some patients I see are actually draining into their bodies the
diseased thoughts of their mind. ~~ Zacharty Bercovitz

Assessing the physical branch of health, alone, is a necessary but insufficient when addressing optimal soul health. We cannot experience radiant health unless we understand not only how the soul directly influences physical health—and how physical health affects the soul, too— but also how problems in any of the other branches of well-being may manifest in the physical body.

Countless theories attempt to explain or understand the mind-body connection. The oldest and most comprehensive that we know of is the practice of Chinese medicine which has existed for over two thousand years. Yet, in Western culture, it is considered an alternative practice to modern medicine. The theory behind Chinese medicine is based on the harmonious interaction of internal entities that regulate overall function. Practitioners of Chinese medicine place little attention on anatomical structures themselves; instead, they focus on identifying the source of the inner disharmony that causes physical illness.

Other authors (Carolyn Myss, Louise Hay, Michael J. Lincoln, J.P. Barral, Debbie Shapiro, Suzanne Scurlock-Durana and others) directly interpret physical illness as related to emotional or psychological concerns. Their texts draw uncanny connections between our physical concerns and those of our psyche. Practitioners who utilize these resources continue to amaze their clients by helping them to make these connections.

The truth is our body "talks" to us in a language that comes directly from the soul. Because our soul's potential is infinite evolution, it wants us to create a healthy and vibrant physical environment to foster its growth. However, our experience of health problems is two-fold. On one hand we either become ill because we aren't listening to cues from our soul and, on the other, contracting an unexpected illness can set the stage for our growth in a new direction. In the former, our soul is trying to get our attention to tell us that we are ignoring important aspects of our lives, while in the latter, an illness can be viewed as a correction of sorts to put our life on a path toward a healthier or more fulfilling way of being. Our conscious response to either scenario is the key to our ability to evolve beyond the situation.

In my own life, my awareness of the mind-body-spirit connection was growing even when I didn't realize it. During my freshman year in high school I developed severe migraines. One day in class, my vision suddenly blurred and, not knowing what was happening, I went home from school only to develop a severe headache and nausea. Episodes like this went on for several years until I started to recognize a pattern. Each migraine started during a very stressful time in my life, and persisted under a combination of stress, sleeplessness, and caffeine intake. When the stress and sleeplessness weren't enough to get my attention, a drink of soda or coffee would throw me over the edge. Thanks to the suggestion of a friend's aunt, I stopped drinking caffeine. The migraines became less frequent, but it wasn't until I monitored my stress and sleeplessness that I was able to eliminate them. I came to realize that I was ignoring the cues from my soul that something was wrong in the way I was living. Once I eliminated what was causing the stress and sleeplessness, my headaches went away. Now, if I experience the signs of a migraine, these symptoms serve as cues to assess and adjust my life in a way that rebalances my own branches of soul health.

The body has its own language. It tells a tale of aches, pains, tensions, stiffness, and illness; however, many choose to ignore what their bodies are telling them and instead allow worse afflictions to undermine their physical health. Suzanne Scurlock-Durana, a cranio-sacral therapist, or body worker, notes that "Being willing to listen to our bodies is the first step in the journey home to ourselves." Many who deny or ignore what is going on inside of their bodies are actually afraid to know their souls. And it can be threatening to those who are unaware, when others who are trained to interpret the body's responses are able to read them like a book.

Several years ago a 50-year-old man entered my psychotherapy practice to deal with life stress. It turned out that he had been having an affair and was deciding whether or not to leave his 30-year marriage. During that initial interview, though, it was very clear to me that he had other issues as well. He had a high-stress personality—one that is commonly called Type A. He was a workaholic, extremely uptight, meticulous about his appearance, and—probably most challenging—he was narcissistic, which manifested in his controlling personality. At the end of that initial session, I asked him if he had any of the following: high blood pressure, tightness in his chest, intestinal problems, constipation, headaches, or hemorrhoids. He stopped with a slightly paranoid tone and asked if I had read his medical chart. He said that he did, in fact, suffer from a long history of all of those symptoms, which had recently intensified.

It was more than clear to me, though not to him, that his physical symptoms were manifestations of lifelong personality traits and habits. He admitted that he had never felt happy, that he always had a difficult time interacting with others, and that his doctors had told him for years to cut down on his stress, which he had refused to do. All along, his soul had been trying to tell him to change his ways, but after years of ignoring its signals, he had developed more intense health problems that were going to be very difficult to turn around. Had he known how to read the messages from his soul sooner, he might have avoided many years of uncomfortable and dangerous physical complaints.

I have many such stories about the mind-body connections that I have explored with clients through my psychotherapy practice.

Because I have also had extensive experience in health and medical settings, physicians and other healthcare workers often send me clients with complicated physical illnesses. On a daily basis, I help clients make the connections between what their bodies are experiencing and what their souls are trying to tell them. People with foot, leg, and hip issues, often have some sort of fear of moving forward in an aspect of their lives. Those with chronic headaches and migraines, tend to over-analyze and to be highly self critical. Patients with breast cancer often have a longstanding need for security or nurturance. Heart problems may arise from a fear of love or a perceived obstacle to love or loving feelings. Intestinal issues usually show up in people who hold on to the past too tightly (constipation) or let go of themselves and their identity too much (diarrhea). Back problems often develop in people who feel overburdened by life and the section of the back that is affected can provide clues as to the kinds and sources of the burdens. The list goes on and on.

Many people think the body is its own entity, separate from all other aspects of their experience as humans. This is not the case. It only takes a little self-awareness to start connecting the dots. When was the last time you were flattened by a cold or flu after having been too busy for your own good? Your soul was trying to get you to slow down. How do you feel after eating or drinking too much? Are you hung over? Guilty? Feeling a little sick? Again, your soul is probably sending the message to exercise moderation both to avoid these after-effects and also to unearth whatever you are avoiding by overdoing it. How often do you listen to your body when it needs a nap? And how aware are you of physical rather than emotional hunger? Physical hunger is your signal to eat, but many eat for reasons other than this but aren't identified as such while eating. Many such bodily cues come with very simple messages, but few people raise their consciousness enough to actually hear the messages and act accordingly. In everything from to day-to-day awareness to a fully developed, long-term understanding of physical concerns, there is much more than meets the eye.

The word "metaphysical" refers to anything beyond or transcending (meta) the physical world (physics) and our powers of direct perception. Metaphysics examines the fundamental nature of reality and being within the world. This branch of philosophy dates from before Aristotle when he first coined the word metaphysics and emphasized what he called the first philosophy, which focuses on the study of 1) being or existence, 2) spiritual or religious issues, and 3) how things relate or interact. Given that our human body wouldn't exist without our soul, and vice versa, we cannot separate the importance of listening to and understanding both, particularly if we hope to evolve as not only individuals, but also as a species.

Because poor physical health threatens our very being, our soul's influence on our physical health is multidimensional. It affects and is affected by all branches of our lives. If we allow our body to be unwell, it can inhibit our ability to evolve in general. And yet, if we unexpectedly become ill, dealing with it in a conscious way can also have a positive effect on other aspects of our health. And whether you face a long-term illness or the need for necessary short-term lifestyle changes, all are connected to your overall radiant health—and to the voice of your soul.

As you read through the remainder of this book, you will become increasingly aware that the other branches of soul health play an integral role in physical health. Although we think of physical health as the primary aspect of health itself, it is the influence of the other aspects that constantly interact to create our overall radiance. One cannot exist without the others.

Look back through the brief questionnaire provided above. Listen for the deepest voice within and its message. Then spend some time thinking about how your health issues or concerns are related to all the other branches of health. Your understanding of the complexity of "whole" or "soul health" will unfold further for you as you read on. But for now, take your own assessment and see what connections you can draw for yourself.

> » What keeps you from taking care of your physical health?

> » What gets in the way of establishing healthier habits?

> » What would need to happen for you to reach a higher level of radiant health?

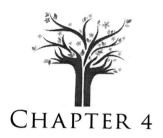

CHAPTER 4

PSYCHOLOGICAL HEALTH:
SYMPTOMS? OR SIGNS FROM YOUR SOUL?

No soul is exempt from a mixture of madness. ~~ Aristotle

While the body is the barometer of the soul, the psyche is its voice. As a psychologist, it is not hard for me to see that when something is not right in a person's world, countless feelings and emotions can erupt to get their attention. These disturbances, whether they relate to general stress, overwhelming circumstances, anxiety, depression, obsession or something even more complicated, are warnings from our soul that something is amiss.

Psychological health has an impact on all other aspects of our well-being, often affecting more than just our physical condition. More and more research is emerging that affirms the mind-body-spirit connection and validates hands-on knowledge that healers and practitioners have used for centuries. Historically, philosophers have spoken about madness and hysteria interfering with the quality of human life, while modern-day scientists are just now recognizing that to separate these aspects of the human condition only serves to confuse it more. So, in many ways we are cycling back to the original understanding that we are whole creatures, not dissectible individuals whose bodies are separate from their psyches and souls.

Given this view of the human condition, the psychological branch of health includes everything from *emotional* concerns such as anxiety, depression, and grief to *perceptual* concerns that include self-esteem, body image, and an overall sense of well-being. In fact, our *perception* of our physical health impacts our emotional health and vice versa, whether accurate or not. Those who are overly anxious about their physical health usually make it worse, while those who dismiss the impact of other branches of well-being often feel discontented but can't identify why. If we fail to hear and understand the soul's message we often manifest physical symptoms instead. This, in effect, sends a louder message from the soul—one which is less easily ignored. Therefore, to experience complete soul health, one must understand that the psyche is often in charge of creating it and sometimes guilty of denying or disregarding it.

MESSAGES TO THE SOUL

Run your fingers through my soul. For once, just once, feel exactly what I feel, believe what I believe, perceive as I perceive, look, experience, examine, and for once; just once, understand. ~~ Unknown

In speaking about the soul, it is important to distinguish feelings from emotions. A feeling is an *affective* state of consciousness, one that can be felt throughout the body depending on what the feeling is. However, an emotion is a *mental* state of consciousness that arises after a feeling or sense is recognized and placed under some sort of judgment about its origin, experience, or potential impact. For example, we may experience a *feeling* that something is not right in our world—a *sense* of anxiety, stress, or discomfort—, but this does not transform into an *emotion* until a judgment is placed on it for how it will affect our lives. We may feel the anxiety arise in our bodies (heart racing, tightness in our chest, sudden flush of heat)—a very normal and healthy reaction in many cases—but then develop scary thoughts about what this will mean for us. The feeling is the alert ("I feel anxious."), and the emotion comes from the judgment we make about the possible impact ("I'm afraid I can't handle this situation."). The sensation of feeling the anxiety is the cue, while the thoughts about the anxious response creates the emotion. Therefore, although many people use the words interchangeably, feelings and emotions serve different purposes in both our human condition and our soul's evolution.

Our soul needs both feelings and emotions in order to evolve. Each is a necessary part of our growth. However, few people are taught to observe their emotions to extract and/or interpret the meaning embedded within them. Instead, we are conditioned by our parents, schooling, and society that emotions are either good or bad. Thus, we either embrace or dismiss them accordingly. The judgments we place on our emotions are a result of several generations before us who lost touch with their souls, and, in many ways, lost touch with their ability to evolve.

When we avoid our feelings, we inhibit or block our soul and its evolution. In doing so, we do an injustice to our greatest ally. This is counterproductive to our growth and stifles our consciousness. Unless we pay attention to our feelings and emotions and deal with them accordingly, our natural voice—our soul—cannot express itself. If something is wrong in our lives, we need the feeling to alert us and we need the emotion to help us tune into the inner voice and tell us what it is and what it means. The purest state of our soul is very peaceful, gentle, loving, and secure. However, when something disrupts this, it is a signal for potential growth, not something to be dismissed. In reality, we wouldn't be feeling something unless there was an opportunity to grow from it in some way. The key is to interpret the feeling and/or emotion instead of ignoring it, rather than bury it beneath our awareness, explain it away, or become absorbed by it as part of the human condition.

Emotional discomfort, then, can actually be a sign that we are losing—or have lost touch with—an awareness of our soul. But this can serve as a catalyst to positive change if we recognize it as such. When we are mired in the human condition, we often disconnect from the soul-based viewpoint that helps us interpret messages embedded within. Instead of gently *observing* what is going on in our world—a response typical of the soul—, we become *absorbed* by it—a reaction inherent to the human condition. These kinds of experiences obscure our power of discernment and dislodge us from the peacefulness of our soul, leaving us less able to make healthy decisions and solve the problems of everyday life.

Essentially, an emotional upsurge is a sign that an important change might be at hand. Much the way a volcanic eruption can signal a subsequent earthquake which naturally shifts the earth's tectonic plates emotional flare-ups can lead to necessary adjustments in various facets of our lives. In many cases the result can enhance our overall soul health. In other words, turmoil can be a platform for the soul's evolution. With each new emotional wound or upset comes the opportunity to evolve beyond it. It can be seen as psychological conditioning, which, instead of blocking the soul, allows it to evolve. By choosing not to *react* to pain or complications in our lives—and instead choosing to *respond* to it— we can learn to see the events of the human condition as opportunities for growth, not obstacles to our well-being. Because we don't generally change without some sort of prompt to do so, our emotions can serve as the catalyst to our evolution. This soul-based stimulation is a natural part of our soul health.

The biggest challenge during times of emotional upset is to recognize crises as opportunities—and then to recognize which branches of soul health need work. In the Chinese written language, the same symbol is used to describe both a crisis and an opportunity; however, the meaning shifts depending on the context. Similarly, emotions can ellicit either a reaction or response depending on our circumstances and how we interpret the emotion.

Although our emotions arise naturally from the human condition, we always long to regain some level of contentment, which is the natural state of the soul. If anything is the death of the soul, it is the refusal to learn life's lessons, choosing instead to deny our feelings rather than work through them.

We all want others to understand us and fully embrace our experiences of the world. We want them to affirm us by hearing and understanding us. But how can they hear us if we don't hear ourselves? How can we embrace the messages of our own soul if we shut our ears to its voice? We don't stand a chance of evolving, let alone living, if we ignore our inner wisdom.

THE HUMAN EXPERIENCE OF EMOTION

Life is marked off on the soul by feelings,
not by dates. ~~ Helen Keller

There's no doubt that emotions are uncomfortable. But they are also uniquely human. Although there is evidence that other species experience at least some basic feelings—sadness, anger and excitement-- humans remain the sole keepers of the vast array of emotions in our world since we place considerably more meaning upon the feelings we experience.

Each emotion holds a unique message. Each translates the voice of our soul into a warning that something is disrupting its contentment either by threatening our truth—the expression of our soul—or by raising a challenge we must face in order to evolve. Either experience causes our soul to bristle, but it does so only to let us know that some sort of growth is on the horizon *if* we welcome the opportunity.

Why else would we have emotion? What other purpose could it serve?

The "fight or flight" response to danger was first described in 1914 by Walter Bradford Cannon, an American physiologist. Cannon theorized that animals react to threats through primal responses such as fighting or fleeing. This concept was later applied to explain ways in which humans reduce stress to a level of homeostasis in which basic needs are safely and satisfyingly met. Homeostasis is now understood to hold polarity, however. In other words, animals and humans may run *away* from something that is a threat, or *toward* something that can restore safety and security.

In a similar way, the soul alerts us through our emotions to our own fight or flight response when it perceives a threat to its integrity. This emotional alarm signifies some sort of danger, one that might elicit a fight to protect our truth or one that lets us know we are fleeing an opportunity to grow. A person's tendency to fight or flee has to do with his or her level of consciousness and desire for growth. Those who are radically conscious are able to *observe* their initial reaction, reflect on their options, and choose an appropriate action intended for growth. Those who are not as deeply aware of their emotional reactions generally remain mired in the fight or flight reaction, either digging themselves deeper into their emotion, or ignoring it altogether by running from it.

Thus, our conscious, reflective response to our emotions is crucial to the vitality of our soul. The more we listen to and honor our feelings and emotions, the more we are able to evolve beyond them and reach new levels of understanding ourselves and the world around us. Our soul itself feels no emotion—it merely uses them to prompt us to grow.

Our soul knows immediately when something threatens its integrity or truth and subsequently initiates an emotional response which we experience as part of our human condition. Given our fight or flight reaction, we must decide whether to move *away* from what threatens us or move *toward* something that can help us. We can best support soul health by continually recognizing and monitoring our reactions to these threats, whether physical, emotional, social and so on. This process helps us decide what needs to be adjusted— removed from or added to our lives— in order to evolve. Recurring emotions can be viewed as reminders that we may be overlooking or avoiding something that would allow us to evolve. Once recognized and understood in terms of balancing the branches of soul health, these emotions generally cease to exist—a sign that you have heard the soul's call and evolved beyond whatever was blocking your evolution.

Perhaps the most obvious example of this is when we place ourselves in the same kinds of situations over and over again and experience the same cycle of emotions as a result. Our repetitive emotions are the sign that something is wrong and that we need to explore why we continue to allow this. The emotion that arises again and again is the sign from our soul to wake up and do what is necessary to change this pattern. If we do not, we create a numbing effect to the soul. We fail to learn the inherent life lesson and in one way or another start the cycle all over again.

Unfortunately, this anesthetizing effect is all too common. The result is not only a lack of growth, but sometimes even a regression. In essence, those who choose not to hear the message behind the emotion have deadened their souls as a result. This creates not only stagnation, but often the resentment of others who do pay attention and move ahead—which of course often causes further emotional sedation. While evolution stimulates more evolution, stagnation stops growth entirely.

Anyone who chooses to move beyond an emotional concern must consciously choose to do so. Most people don't enjoy dealing with painful feelings, but choosing to evolve beyond them—to identify their cause, interpret their message, and find a way to resolve them—takes far less energy than the drain it places on the soul ,and consequently on overall soul health, to ignore them. This is where psychological conditions such as anxiety and depression come in. These symptoms of the soul are often a compilation of unattended or misunderstood emotions. For example, anxiety is the synthesis of both feelings and emotions—our initial response as well as the judgment or meaning we place on that reaction—, and often erupts as soon as a conditioned response to fear is initiated. The experience of anxiety depends on the meaning we place upon it in relation to our experiences within the human condition. When a person ignores an emotion and only attends to the feeling, as is often done when a person takes psychotropic medications without engaging in psychotherapy, no evolution beyond the anxiety will occur. There will only be symptom relief. But if, in addition to medications (which are sometimes necessary for biological reasons), the person comes to an understanding of the anxiety through psychotherapy and other methods, it is often possible to eliminate the anxiety altogether, thus evolving beyond it.

Methods such as Cognitive Behavioral Therapy can be part of this process, but they are insufficient in ameliorating of the condition at the soul level. It is not just a matter of making the symptoms go away; instead, it is more about retrieving the message from the soul that is there to stimulate growth. When I was suffering from migraines, I had to understand my stress, and the impact it had on my health, in order to make the changes that would eliminate the stress altogether. It is challenging in our world to understand that we need our emotions in order to grow. However, there is no cure for a sad soul but to listen to its needs and take steps needed to improve soul health.

We all seek some level of peace and contentment—the most natural state of our soul. We intuitively know what our homeostasis feels like, and we especially crave this contented state in the midst of emotional turmoil. The trick is to recognize that our emotions are catalysts for growth rather than nuisances to be ignored. This is the key to our soul's evolution. Then we must learn how to use feelings and emotions for our benefit.

LISTENING WITHIN

Whenever anyone has offended me, I try to raise my soul so high that the offense cannot reach it. ~~ Rene Descartes

Because human emotions and other aspects of psychological health are so complex, we must learn to extract and understand the meaning embedded in each so that we can learn to release it and move on. Only then do we evolve. Only then do we become students of the soul rather than victims of the human condition.

In my psychotherapy practice, I have come to realize that it is necessary but insufficient to heal from a painful event. The added essential element in the therapeutic relationship is a commitment to our evolution. Relief from emotional symptoms is not my goal in working with clients; freeing them to evolve is. Instead of working with "victims," I create an environment for interpretation and growth. As a result, my clients build an indestructible toolbox for managing their life's challenges. Their only responsibility thereafter is to maintain the consciousness that their evolutionary process requires, even beyond therapy.

The psychological branch of soul health encompasses many dimensions. All emotions and psychological concerns are a part of it, as they are part of the human condition. In describing troublesome emotions, we use a variety of terms to capture our sense of not being at peace. Sadness, depression, grief, anxiety, anger, and so on all characterize our human experience, but do not describe the soul. So, when our psyche is unhealthy we suffer from a *dis*-ease of the soul; our soul is dis-contented. Our emotions are not just symptoms to be ignored but strong signals that we need to make changes in our lives.

In his Pulitzer Prize winning book *Travels with Charley: In Search of America*, John Steinbeck wrote, "A sad soul can kill quicker, far quicker, than a germ." Through his own dark nights, he recognized that to become engulfed in emotion is to become immobilized by the human condition.

So how do we use an awareness of our psychological health to face our challenges rather than run away from them? Take the following questionnaire, but in doing so, explore what you think your soul is trying to tell you through each of the symptoms—or, better —signs you recognize. Understand that each emotional concern or challenge is nothing more than a prompt, an opportunity to enhance the health of your soul through conscious searching and understanding.

QUESTIONNAIRE FOR THE PSYCHOLOGICAL BRANCH OF HEALTH

On a scale of 1 to 10, rate the level of your health within each area described. A 10 describes optimal, radiant health, while a 1 describes an almost complete lack of health within the given aspect of the psychological branch. Remember, this questionnaire is designed to create a roadmap to overall radiant health. It is not meant to overwhelm you.

Stress

1. _____ I recognize and can acknowledge the stressors in my life.
2. _____ I know how to manage my stress in ways that enhance my overall health.
3. _____ I am open to professional help when stress overwhelms me.
4. _____ I proactively engage in activities that help to reduce or prevent stress.
5. _____ I am aware of how my emotional stress affects other aspects or branches of my health.

Psychological Concerns

1. _____ I am free of depression and ongoing sad thoughts.
2. _____ I am free of worrisome or anxious thoughts.
3. _____ I have good overall psychological health.
4. _____ I know when and how to seek professional help for any psychological concern.
5. _____ I willingly seek professional help for psychological concerns.
6. _____ I engage in proactive behaviors that enhance my psychological health.
7. _____ I can identify and express the full range of my emotions.
8. _____ I handle my emotions in a healthy way.
9. _____ I concentrate well on tasks I undertake.
10. _____ I face my fears.

Self-Esteem

1. _____ I like myself.
2. _____ I know and accept my worth.
3. _____ I have only positive thoughts about myself.
4. _____ I know and accept who I am.
5. _____ I am self-confident.
6. _____ I am successful in most areas of my life.

Self-Awareness

1. _____ I know my strengths and weaknesses.
2. _____ I can accurately describe how I impact others.
3. _____ I am generally self-aware.
4. _____ I am able to identify the source of my emotional concerns quickly.
5. _____ I actively work to be self-aware and to learn about myself.
6. _____ I have healthy emotional boundaries.

Perceptions

1. _____ I have a positive outlook on life.
2. _____ I am open to all that life has to offer.
3. _____ I can accurately describe things that happen around me.
4. _____ I see the world as a good place.
5. _____ I understand and accept that people have ideas and beliefs different from my own.
6. _____ My perceptions of myself match what others think of me.

Much like taking the Questionnaire for the Physical Branch of Health, you may have recognized some inner stirrings for certain questions. Even in the twenty-first century, we are still shy about admitting challenges to our psychological health. That is unfortunate, given that our psychological health is the voice of our soul. Out of all of the branches of health, we judge ourselves the most on the psychological branch. Somehow we think we should portray a clean bill of psychological health despite the constant challenges of the complex, troubled world around us.

STRESS

Who doesn't have stress? Who feels a sense of peace all the time? Why do we assume we are inadequate or at fault if we admit to a difficult feeling or emotion? And what makes us think that our lives would be fulfilled if we didn't experience the ups and downs of the human condition?

Stress is the sense that our internal resources cannot overcome our external stressors. Instead of taking an inner inventory of our ability to cope, most people, when subjected to stress, tend to think that they don't have what it takes to withstand it.

However, stress is essential to life. It motivates us and initiates life-sustaining behavior. It is the natural reaction when our bodies, psyches, or souls are threatened in some way. The only problem is that many people 'cope' in the wrong direction. Instead of facing stress head-on, they hide behind their vices, seeking a short-term diversion from their emotional strain.

But stress can motivate us to grow if we understand that we can escape our discomfort permanently. Our soul seeks inner peace, and when this is disrupted, it initiates our stress response in an effort to prompt us to find a way of regaining a comfortable balance.

» How do you handle stress?

>   » How could you handle it better?

>   » What do you perceive as your biggest stressors?

>   » Which other branches of your soul health contribute to your stress?

PSYCHOLOGICAL CONCERNS

Somehow we have created a skewed view of what life is all about. In the book *The Art of Happiness,* the Dalai Lama emphasizes that western cultures have come to believe we are supposed to be happy at all times. But he says happiness is a way of *thinking*, not a way of *being*, and the things that make us unhappy are there to be observed, not reacted to. Although he did not use the terms, he was speaking of the psychological branch of soul health.

We do many things to make us happy, but few last more than a short time. We shop, eat, drink, gamble, have sex, play games, sit at the computer, work, and many other things just to avoid being unhappy. And yet, instead of addressing the problem, we are stifling our ability to evolve beyond it.

As discussed, our psychological discomfort is often a cue or symptom of the soul, and these are often related strongly to other branches of soul health and their impact on our psychological health.

>   » What are your primary psychological concerns?

>   » How do they affect your overall sense of radiant living?

>   » What would life feel like without these concerns?

SELF-ESTEEM

How long has it been since you truly liked—or even loved—yourself? This is a tough question for most. Many people have never liked themselves, let alone felt they measured up to the expectations of others.

As mentioned earlier, to know yourself is to know your soul. But many people are terrified to truly know themselves because they are afraid they will not like what they see. To find confidence and satisfaction in oneself is often seen as egotistical, but only those who truly know and accept themselves are able to reach optimal health—the most complete and radiant expression of the soul. True knowledge and acceptance of self, regardless of what others may think, creates pure self-love rather than dislike or judgment. When we assess ourselves from the *outside in* —basing our worth on what others may think—we jeopardize the health of our soul. However, when we base our worth on what feels right to *us*,—living from the *inside out*— we become better acquainted with our soul. The former describes self-esteem, while the later describes the soul's integrity. The challenge is to find enough peace within oneself to satisfy the soul, which promotes our ultimate contentment.

Our soul is what it is. It makes no judgments; it only prompts us to provide what it wants or needs to survive and thrive. The soul has no ego, only acceptance and unconditional encouragement from within, and so it guides us toward what everyone deserves—optimal health.

» In what ways do you struggle with self-esteem?

» Are you afraid to acknowledge your worth? Your greatness?

» How do your feelings about yourself affect your health?

SELF-AWARENESS

People often become self-absorbed and less aware of others when they feel bad emotionally, but they don't always know how to change this.

It may seem like a cliché', but awareness really is the first step toward improving all areas of life. If you never acknowledge your discomfort, then you will never change. In essence, your level of awareness—and ultimately your radical consciousness— is proportionate to your experience of soul health. The more you become aware, the more you are likely to honor your soul. The more you honor your soul, the more you grow or evolve. Those who remain unaware or unconscious also remain stagnant in their experience of life, not to mention in their soul's evolution.

> » What are you most aware of in your well-being today?

> » What have you become more aware of by reading this book so far?

> » In what ways have you avoided self-awareness?

PERCEPTIONS

The way we look at life is also the way we approach it. If we see the world through dark glasses, then we will live with less light. So our psychological health depends entirely on how we perceive ourselves and the world around us.

Our soul requires an optimistic outlook in order to grow. Although human life is not all rosy, it is our hope and anticipation that we can improve it that allows us to evolve beyond our old ways. Without this positive outlook we dampen our soul and the darkness of the human condition takes hold.

»   How do you look at the world?

»   What are your expectations for experiencing a happier and
    healthier life?

»   What do you need to work on or change in order to brighten
    your perceptions?

Psychological health is a complex part of our overall radiant health.
However, as in other branches of health, our radical consciousness of
what we need in this area is essential to finding the fullest expression
of health, which is soul health.

BECOMING A STUDENT OF THE SOUL

*When you do things from your soul you feel a river
moving in you, a joy. When action comes from
another section the feeling disappears.* ~~ Rumi

There are two core emotions that humans experience: love and
fear. All others are simply variations on one or the other. However,
one is purely soul-based, while the other is most reflective of the
human condition. It's not difficult to guess which is which.

Love, of course, is a soul-based emotion. It is the return to our
most natural state of being—one we all desire. This is what we strive
for, hope and yearn for. All sense of joy, compassion, peacefulness,
generosity, unconditionality, gratitude, ease, hope, empathy, and all
other positively charged emotions are *love*-based, and as a result are
also *soul*-based. When we remain in the soul, life feels good. When
we deviate from our soul, we feel bad.

We feel fearful when we move away from the love and peacefulness
of our soul. Through our fear, we *react* instead of reflect and *respond.*
Our daily lives and cares take over, anxiety rises up, and instead of

observing our situations and reflecting on how to regain this sense of peace we react through the fear of never reaching that state again. We don't take the time to recognize that, in that moment, fear is the voice of our soul urging us to learn from our troubles to find the path back to peace. If we aren't alert to this voice we may sink further into the fear and become more deeply mired in the human condition.

Anger, sadness, resentment, frustration, worry, irritation and so on are all symptoms of the human condition, yet they are initiated by the soul for the sake of our evolution—for the sake of re-establishing peace in some way. All fear-based emotions are negatively charged, but they serve as vital cues that something in our lives requires work. Anger represents a fear of not protecting the integrity of our soul in one way or another. Sadness usually indicates a fear of losing—or having lost— something that is dear to us. Resentment is an indication that we allowed something to happen that had a negative impact our soul. Worry represents the fear that our resources aren't enough to overcome troubling events or situations. Irritation typically represents a mirror in something we have seen in someone else that we need to work on or change within ourselves.

In fact, our emotions have nothing to do with another person. They have everything to do with our soul. Our reactions come from a lifetime of accumulated experiences in the human condition, many of which don't work toward our sense of well-being. Recurrent emotions, then, are the red flags that alert us to something we are to learn about ourselves, not something that someone or something has done to us. The purpose of life—and our experience of emotion— is to expand our awareness, which means to expand or evolve our souls. Our emotions offer the chance to protect the health or integrity of our soul if we reflect on them and make the necessary changes in our lives or perceptions. Though they can be fierce and arise without warning, once a person accepts these difficult emotions as possibilities for growth, he or she can *respond* from the soul instead of *react* from the human condition. A soul response is the only way to evolve beyond any emotional reaction.

As mentioned earlier, depression and anxiety are complex symptoms of the soul. Although we may be biologically predisposed to them, depression and anxiety appear only in response to troublesome experiences. Even if we have a genetic link to certain psychological issues, these will never emerge unless our experiences trigger them. It is inaccurate to say that these conditions are strictly medical—which is why psychotropic medications do little to fix the situation, although they may offer relief from uncomfortable symptoms. Disregarding the human condition's role in these psychological conditions only disregards the voice of the soul. One does not become depressed without experiencing something that challenges one or more branches of their well-being. One does not become anxious without an anxiety-provoking event. The soul speaks whether we like it or not, and sometimes it has to yell.

As you can see, all emotions, no matter how perplexing at first, are quite logical in nature. Something that makes you feel empty is a sign that you need to fill something up. Something that makes you angry and resentful suggests that you allowed things to happen that went against your soul. And sometimes our emotions have to feel overwhelming in order to guide us to a subtle sense of peace.

In essence, all emotions are valid indicators that something is threatening your soul's integrity—your soul health. These indicators could apply to any or all branches of soul health, depending on the emotion that is triggered. Much as the body has its own language, the language of emotions is interpretable depending on your level of consciousness. Many people don't believe they have a right to feelings and emotions, particularly if they come from families or cultures that choose to dismiss them. However, sometimes a sense of invalidation can teach us greater self-respect in the long run as a soul-based and loving movement toward our evolution. Choosing to learn about our souls through our feelings and emotions is a critical step in our growth as human beings.

To become a student of the soul means to embrace our feelings and emotions as key elements in our growth. As we listen to—and heed— the voice of our soul, we can begin to partner with our greatest ally to promote optimal health. When we create this key alliance with our soul—our inner wisdom—we create a joint effort not only toward healing from our emotional wounds, but toward our evolution beyond them.

Reaching radical consciousness of emotions means you are mastering the language of your soul. You have earned your advanced degree in understanding the human condition and consciously committing to your evolution. Strangely enough, once you get the hang of it, the work not only becomes easier, but also more light-hearted and amusing along the way. You learn to laugh with your soul each time you see that you are reacting to your old habits of the human condition. You give yourself a break and move through difficult emotions much more quickly and easily.

Which do you want—to heal a wound or to evolve beyond it? Even the question elicits a radiant response! There is something inexplicably exciting about feeling like you can outgrow your old skin. There is an energy behind it—a momentum—that once begun doesn't want to stop. This is the soul's radiance urging you toward your evolution.

Emotions carry energy. And because everything around us consists of energy at the most basic level, it stands to reason that we are most attracted to things that make us feel light. Moths to a flame are drawn to an external light they seek as their own, and die in the pursuit of reaching it. We, however, are able to pursue our inner light, and our emotions are nothing more than a signal pointing the way to find it. But unfortunately, we get mired in the human condition and buried in our emotions instead of using them to find and return to our inner radiance. We all know people who emit a simple yet desirable brightness or light. Much like the moth, we are instinctively drawn to these individuals and want to catch a bit of what they seem to have and that which we seem to lack. This light is for our taking, but we must find it within ourselves.

In essence, we are all beings of light. We are meant to emit brighter and brighter radiance if we allow ourselves. This happens only if we evolve, and we evolve only if we use the voice of our soul to do so. If we do not, our lights dim and we just fizzle out. There is no more light and no sign of growth.

SECRETS OF THE SOUL

Our psychological health, like our physical health, depends on our willingness and ability to create optimal conditions. Without these conditions, we cannot fully evolve. The following tips and exercises will help you both assess the psychological branch of soul health and also set the wheels in motion for experiencing your soul's ultimate peace and radiance.

1. First, know that change doesn't come without inconvenience. Yes, it can be uncomfortable to assess and enhance your psychological branch of health. But the result is what we are all looking for—inner joy and peace. We learn to experience this state of being regardless of our circumstances if we honor the messages from our soul. We need to master its language.

2. In general, we create change only when we get tired enough of ourselves or our situations. We can talk about changing for years and even decades, but until we get fed up, we tend to remain stuck. Still, these in-between times can be very important to our evolution. Kristin Jongen captures the essence of this through her artwork: "It's in the in-between

that the real magic happens... the seeds are planted...the roots take hold...and we blossom into who we were meant to be." Even when we feel mired in the human condition, we still have the option to learn about ourselves. These seemingly stagnant times are often incubation periods for our soul's next phase of development. Sometimes we need to simply wait in our discomfort for a while in order to know which direction to turn. Seeking radical consciousness of your soul during these times can set the stage for greater understanding as well as growth beyond the situation.

3. Once you change a particular aspect of how you see or understand yourself, and you feel the benefit to your soul health, you generally don't want to stop. There is something inherently motivating and almost addictive about your soul's growth. One insight seems to lead to the next. All we need is to give ourselves permission to work on our emotional health—and an occasional nudge (if our soul hasn't already done so!). Many of my clients feel this compulsion toward their soul's overall health once they start the process. Once a student of the soul, always a student of the soul!

4. Validate but don't perseverate. In other words, acknowledge your feelings and emotions, but don't get stuck in them. They are simply messages. Because they can be seductive — pulling us to feel and learn about them more deeply—, we must learn to step back and observe them instead of being absorbed by them. If we allow ourselves to become ruled by our emotions—our human condition—, we will not evolve.

5. As you review the Questionnaire for the Psychological Branch of Soul Health, listen for what your soul is trying to tell you. Yes, some of it may be difficult to hear and even more difficult

to want to change. But at least hear the message. Then set the path toward cleaning out and/or filling up whatever will enhance your psychological health. Whether this requires a commitment to seeking professional guidance, reading or journaling on your own, or simply observing your situation, your soul will eventually grow lighter.

» What have you been avoiding in the psychological branch of your health?

» What old thoughts, beliefs, or feelings do you need to observe and reflect on in order to evolve beyond them?

» In what ways have you allowed yourself to be controlled by your emotions instead of becoming a student of your soul?

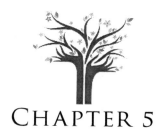

CHAPTER 5

SOCIAL HEALTH:
SOUL TO SOUL RELATIONS

*We are all dependent on one another, every soul
of us on earth.* ~~ George Bernard Shaw

Humans are pack animals—we are meant to be with people. No matter how 'independent' we think we are, we still depend on those around us for at least some things, and we obviously wouldn't have been brought into the world without the help of others. In most cases we could not survive, let alone thrive without the help of parents or other caregivers, teachers, friends, neighbors, pets and others. What makes the world go around is our connection with others and the sense of community we receive through these interactions.

All of our relationships can have a direct impact on soul health. If I were to guess, I'd say nearly 90 percent of people come to therapy because of their relationships with others in their lives. Depression, anxiety, grief, adjustment, low self-esteem, job stress, body image, weight-related concerns, physical injuries, traumatic events, anger management, abuse, and even some ongoing physical health concerns can be attributed to either present-day interactions with others or to the ideas, values or beliefs we were taught as children.

The social branch of soul health encompasses all the relationships we have in our lives. This chapter discusses the many types of connections we have with other people, not only those close to us, but also others we may see less frequently—store clerks, drycleaners, mail carriers, receptionists, pharmacists, manicurists, massage therapists, hair stylists, and even coffee baristas. Many people, including me, also consider pets and other animals to be significant contributors to our overall social health. No matter how connected we are to those who appear regularly in our lives, they are all part of our personal flock.

Take note that this chapter discusses the types of relationships that contribute to our overall soul health, while the next chapter on the interpersonal branch of health discusses the specific dynamics of each type of relationship.

OUR SOUL TO SOUL RELATIONS

True intimacy is the opening of one soul to another. No gift on earth could compare with it, for it touches us more profoundly than our imagination can envision. When two people share their lives, freely, openly, without reservation, it is as if each had become complete. ~~ Robert Sexton

The company we keep has a lot to do with how we feel at the soul level. We need more than just "warm bodies" in our lives; we need connection to others that makes us feel complete. And yet, it is often our quest for completeness from others, and not from within that causes our discontent, and thus, undermines our soul health. We may create a large social network, but seldom considering how these connections might affect our soul.

The social branch of soul health should enhance all the other branches, although this is not always the case. Our relationships either affirm or diminish our lives and our soul health. As mentioned in the previous chapter, people seem to carry an energy or light within them, and this can be bright or dim, positive or negative depending on the health of their soul. Spending time with people who are life-affirming tends to leave you feeling positive, joyful, and charged; these relationships have a "life-giving" quality. Those who are life-diminished tend to leave you feeling negative, depleted and drained and take on a "life-taking" quality while in their presence. Life-affirmers have healthier and brighter souls. Life diminishers' soul health is compromised, leaving them with a dimmer or darker presence. It is not uncommon for those with more damaged souls to be drawn to those who are healthier, though this can create a somewhat parasitic relationship in which the darker would draw upon the light in order to survive. It is somewhat like charging a depleted battery—these people need others' light to feel alive.

In contrast, relationships between life-affirmers are very healthy and mutually beneficial. These connections are non dramatic, simple, and easy. Except for casual discussion about daily matters, and normal adjustments to life, these unions continue to provide ongoing, life-sustaining support for both people. Both parties accept when circumstances change, crises arise, and beliefs shift and both work together to maintain the health of the relationship. It is the constellation of all our relationships that allows us to move through personal imbalances and changes and regain our ability to grow and thrive.

Following are descriptions of the types of social connections we usually make. As you read through them, take note of whether you feel they are life-affirming or life-diminishing. This will help you assess your social branch of health. Later in the chapter you will be offered a Questionnaire for the Social Branch of Health which will assess the quality of your relationships.

FAMILY RELATIONS

Your soul is a dark forest. But the trees are of a particular species, they are genealogical trees. ~~ Marcel Proust

A standard joke for many people is that they tolerate family holidays so that they can enjoy the rest of the year. Once we arrive in this world, we are generally stuck with the families into which we were born. In cases of neglect, abuse, or some other tragedy, this may not be the case. Whether we have a large or small family, one or more parents (including step-parents, adoptive parents, or foster parents), siblings (including step-siblings and half-siblings), grandparents, aunts, uncles, or cousins, the influence family has on us—both positive and negative—is lifelong. Research clearly indicates that a sense of a healthy family community not only extends our lifespan, but also contributes to better overall health and wellness.

Like many things in our evolving life, family structure has changed significantly over the last several decades. "Family" has come to mean different things to different people. The following list is a compilation of descriptions for family from several sociologists:

Nuclear Family—the previously traditional idea of family: husband, wife, and one or more biological or adopted children.

Single-Parent Family—one parent with one or more biological or adopted children.

Blended Family—a couple and one or more children from previous relationships.

Common Law—a couple who is not officially married but have lived together long enough to meet criteria for legal partnership; may or may not have children.

Childless Family—a married or unmarried couple without children.

Extended Family—includes, along with one or more parents and their children, grandparents, aunts, uncles, cousins and all other blood relatives; may or not live in the same household.

Gay Family—same-sex couple who may or may not have children, and may be legally married.

Because of our changing times, many people now have an even broader idea of what family means to them. Close friends, spiritual communities, and pets are now often considered part of a person's family depending on how the individuals define the term for themselves.

FRIENDSHIPS

A true friend is one soul in two bodies. ~~ Aristotle

No one can deny the power of a strong friendship except those who have never had one. Everyone has different needs and comfort levels for the non-family relationships in their lives. Research regarding the positive impact of friendships is extensive in the sociological literature. Among other things, friends abate loneliness, enhance a sense of kinship, and help each other maximize both emotional and physical health.

In their book *Rethinking Friendship*, authors Liz Spencer and Ray Pahl describe the following types of friendly connections:

Associates—those who share common activities like hobbies and sports.

Useful Contacts—those who share information and advice whether for career or other purposes.

Favor Friends—those who help each other in a functional, but not an emotional manner.

Fun Friends—those who socialize together but don't offer deep emotional support.

Helpmates—friends who offer both favors and fun but little emotional support.

Comforters —similar to helpmates, but with some emotional support.

Confidants—those who share personal information with each other but aren't always in a position to offer practical help (i.e., if they live far away).

Soul mates—those who display all of the elements listed above.

Whether a person has one or all of these types of friendships, the evidence clearly shows that it is important to our soul health to cultivate relationships of this kind. As previously noted, many people consider friends to be a vital part of their family network, which enhances your soul health.

LOVE RELATIONS

Love is the fire that ignites the passion in my soul. ~~ Unknown

There's nothing like a romantic relationship to make your heart go pitter-patter. But in many cases these unions can also negatively impact your soul health. In *Colors of Love*, J. A. Lee defined six varieties of love-based relationships.

Eros—romantic, passionate love and the belief that love is life's most important quality. The search for a lifelong, sexually-satisfying commitment or ideal love typifies this kind of relationship.

Ludus—uncommitted relationships that often involve lying and game-playing. People who prefer this type of relationship usually make many sexual conquests without commitment.

Storge (pronounced store-gay) —slow developing, friendship-based love. Activity-based relationship, often resulting in a long-term relationship in which sex might or might not be intense or passionate.

Pragma—pragmatic, practical, mutually beneficial relationship that may be unromantic. Sex is often a technical matter necessary only for producing children.

Mania—an obsessive or possessive type of love that is jealous and extreme. May involve acts that seem crazy, or overly intense.

Agape (pronounced a-ga-pay)—based on a gentle, care-giving type of love that is not concerned with the self. It is relatively rare and typifies someone like Mother Teresa's in her unconditional love for impoverished people.

As noted, love relationships can provide us with passion, but not necessarily soul health. However, our love relationships often provide important experiences from which we can evolve, whether from staying in them or choosing to get out of them. The dynamics—healthy and not—that we learn as a result of our love relationships often stem from our early interactions with our primary caregivers.

These will be discussed further in the next chapter. For now, just note whether your love relationships have been more life-affirming or life-diminishing.

Peripheral Relationships

One may have a blazing hearth in one's soul and yet no one ever come to sit by it. Passersby see only a wisp of smoke from the chimney and continue on the way. ~~ Vincent Van Gogh

We all encounter people in our daily lives who affect us in some way but without intimate ties. In her book *Growing Together*, author Karen Fingerman says that these relationships tend to link us to larger social structures and to provide opportunities for cultural experiences, novel stimulation, exploration of our identities, and brief social support. Peripheral ties arise in all aspects of daily life. They can help us acquire skills we might not get through our families or friends and also present us with new ideas to assimilate about the world in general. Fingerman calls these acquaintances consequential strangers and notes that each has its own impact on our lives.

You probably have many of the following peripheral relationships in your life: neighbors, co-workers, classmates, store clerks, drycleaners, bookkeepers or accountants, cleaning staff, mail carriers, restaurant hosts and wait staff, coffee baristas, bartenders, bank tellers, mechanics, fitness instructors, trash and recycling collectors, public safety officers, child care workers, landscapers and lawn mowers. Of course many more exist, but by now you get the idea that our social branch of health extends far beyond our immediate contacts. All of these contacts affect our social branch of health, and without them our experience of soul health would be greatly reduced.

PETS AND OTHER ANIMALS

Until one has loved an animal, a part of one's soul
remains un-awakened. ~~ Anatole France

I would be remiss to not mention the importance of animals in our social network, particularly with the booming merchandise market aimed specifically at pet lovers. It is clear that our society values pets to the point where many consider them key components of their social branch of health. The National Humane Society reports that 62 percent of U.S. homes have at least one pet (39 percent own at least one dog, 33 percent have at least one cat, and the rest have a mixture of horses, fish, birds, reptiles, and other small animals). Research demonstrates that owning pets can reduce a person's stress, blood pressure, heart rate, depression, anxiety, loneliness, and other issues pertaining to soul health. Many people treat their animals as family members, and a loss of one can be devastating, bringing on as much or more grief as the death of a human loved one.

THE SOUL'S SOCIAL PLAYGROUND

Life is the soul's nursery--its training place for the destinies
of eternity. ~~ William Makepeace Thackeray

As you can see, our social network extends far beyond those with whom we share a genetic link. Our ability to connect with a variety of people and animals is integral not only to our soul's development, but also to maintaining and advancing its health and evolution.

So, who are the people in our lives, really? Why are our bonds with them important? And what can they do for soul health and evolution?

Many have heard of soul mates and assume these relationships only apply to romantic connections. The term dates back to Greek mythology and a story that our ancestors actually had two heads and four arms. After offending the gods, they were split in two and condemned to spend the rest of their lives searching for their other half—their soul mate. Many spiritual traditions subscribe to the idea that, through reincarnation, soul mates travel through many lives together, offering each other ongoing lessons to aid in their soul's evolution. Original books of the Bible are even said to have contained texts that alluded to past lives, but modern editions no longer include these.

Essentially, every individual who has a significant impact on our lives can be considered a soul mate, no longer limiting these connections to romantic love alone. Each is a person from whom we can learn something that will help us grow, and who remains supportive as we do so. An expanded conceptualization is warranted, given how many kinds of encounters can help us profoundly. Several types of soul mates have been described in spiritual literature:

Twin Flame Soul Mates—This type of union is the most commonly thought of—the one we are all searching for. This kind of romantic match is our divine mate, whom we recognize through an extremely strong chemistry and attraction, uncanny similarities, and yet enough differences that once we find each other we feel balanced and complete. Many believe there is only one twin flame soul for each of us and that few of us actually find the one we're meant for.

Twin Souls—Separate from a romantic relationship are soul twins, our closest friends or family—the people with whom we instinctively feel a strong affinity to and likeness. We share such powerful emotional bonds with them that we feel a sense of confidence, trust, and understanding that goes beyond words. These are the folks who seem to know when something is wrong in our world even without talking, and with whom we remain deeply connected even over great distance and extended time apart.

Companion Soul Mates—These are the individuals we encounter throughout life who make more than just a cursory impact on our lives. They are our friends and other associates who help us to attain our life's goals through ongoing encouragement and unconditional support. These individuals may come and go in our lives, but they leave lasting impressions.

Teacher Soul Mates—Whether we like it or not, there are people who enter our Lives whom we may or may not like, but who provide us with difficulties, challenges, and opportunities to grow. They have a profound impact on us, sometimes catastrophically, leaving us no choice but to change the course of our life in some way—desired or not. Some call these individuals Master Teachers if they create an ongoing series of challenges to our worlds, through means we would never choose ourselves and which we might initially resist. We often see such a person as our nemesis because of our adversarial interactions with them. But they are there to lead us to key lessons about ourselves and guide us—often reluctantly—into overcoming or evolving beyond their often infuriating behavior. Recognizing the lessons these people are providing is the tough part.

Keep in mind that regardless of the type of person that enters your life, all are here to help you grow or evolve in one way or another. This soul group may push our buttons as well as support our most valiant efforts, but in any case, these people exist for a reason. Without them, our lives would be empty and our souls would not have the opportunity to thrive.

When we think of the people in our lives as key players in our life's script—one which might be altered or re-written depending on whether we choose to evolve—, we gain insight into their role in our human condition. Sometimes it takes great restraint not to react, as if someone is doing something *to* us, rather than respond from the soul, by recognizing that the interchange is happening *for* us as part of our evolution. This takes some objectivity, but once people adopt this approach, they can choose more effective and life-affirming responses. Too many of us fall victim to these interchanges and relationships, not realizing we can choose to rise above them and avoid an emotional wound.

Though all social connections are important to our soul's growth, when healthy souls unite with other healthy souls, we reach our greatest potential for radiant health.

Take the following questionnaire to assess your social health more fully.

QUESTIONNAIRE FOR THE SOCIAL BRANCH OF HEALTH

On a scale of 1 to 10, rate the level of your health within each area described. A 10 describes optimal, radiant health, while a 1 describes an almost complete lack of health within the given aspect of the social branch. Remember, this questionnaire is designed to create a roadmap to overall radiant health. It is not meant to overwhelm you.

Social Contacts

1. _____ I have enough social support.
2. _____ I have close friends.
3. _____ I am close to my family.
4. _____ Pets are an important part of my social network.
5. _____ I know the names of my neighbors.
6. _____ I enjoy my co-workers and/or fellow students.
7. _____ I am often around like-minded people.
8. _____ I am generally friendly toward others.
9. _____ I develop new relationships easily.
10. _____ I am satisfied with the number of people in my life.
11. _____ I am aware of how my relationships affect other aspects or branches of health.

Time

1. _____ I spend enough time with friends and family.
2. _____ I socialize with friends at least once a week.
3. _____ I live close enough to family.
4. _____ I look forward to spending time with friends and family.
5. _____ I talk frequently with my friends.
6. _____ I talk frequently with my family.
7. _____ I have at least one friend who lives in my town or city.

Quality

1. _____ I like the people in my life.
2. _____ I share many interests with the people in my life.
3. _____ I feel safe and at ease in my friendships and relationships.
4. _____ I value the many of the same things as my friends and vice versa.
5. _____ I feel proud to be friends with those in my life.
6. _____ I feel proud to be part of my family.
7. _____ My friends know who I really am.
8. _____ My family knows who I really am.
9. _____ I only spend time with people who are healthy for me.

Relationship with Self

1. _____ I enjoy spending time alone.
2. _____ I know when I need time alone.
3. _____ I know when I need time with others.
4. _____ I have interests that can be done alone as well as with others.
5. _____ I don't generally get lonely.
6. _____ I am a healthy influence for those in my life.

The social branch of health includes the number and types of contacts we have, the amount of time we spend with each, the quality or richness of our relationships with others, as well as the relationship we have with our self. It goes without saying that we need others in order to survive, but we also need them in order to grow or evolve. We also need our pack, tribe, or soul group to build community and feel a sense of belonging. Without this, our evolution is delayed or even stopped. The next chapter will explore how the characteristics or dynamics of our soul group also impact our overall soul health.

Getting To Know Your Own Soul

As you probably noticed, the Questionnaire for the Social Branch of Health inquires not only about your relationships with others, but also about the one you have with yourself. Few people stop to consider whether they treat themselves the way they would treat others—and few do! We tend to be much more negative and harsh with ourselves than with others. We would never say the negative things to others that we say to ourselves. We often protect and help others before taking care of own lives, health, or well-being. We put friends, family, and even pets before our own interest, and sometimes even attend to our peripheral relationships before we consider our own needs. However, creating and maintaining a healthy relationship with our soul is the only path to soul health. Without it, we will fail to evolve.

In essence, the less you know about yourself and the less you honor what you do know, the poorer your soul health will be. Instead of feeling vibrantly alive, you will feel 'wilty' or burdened overall.

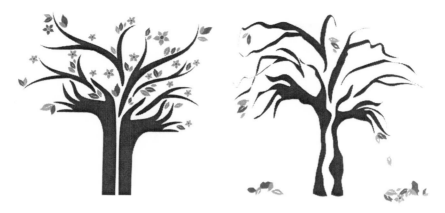

In my experience, most people who enter therapy don't really feel like they know who they are, which leads me to believe that many people outside of therapy likely don't either. The lack of awareness or consciousness about self is striking in the world at large. However, it is often the case that one must *lose* one self—lose touch with our soul—in order to truly find oneself—to recognize the need to reconnect more deeply. In other words, we sometimes need to feel bad enough in order to do something to change or improve our lives. Understanding the social branch of soul health creates not only a stronger awareness of the connections you have with others, but also a more conscious connection with your soul.

The next chapter will explore the basic qualities that describe a healthy interpersonal connection with others. As you read the chapter, consider 1) whether your social connections reflect these qualities, and 2) whether your relationship with *you* does as well.

> » How did I develop my ideas about who is healthy to have in my life?

> » Which of your relationships are life-affirming? Life-diminishing?

» Do you treat yourself as you would your closest friend or family member?

» Can you identify which type of relationship you have with each person in your life?

» What is required to create a healthier relationship with *you*?

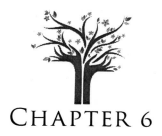

CHAPTER 6

INTERPERSONAL HEALTH:
CREATING CONSCIOUS CONNECTIONS

*Blessed is the influence of one true, loving human
soul on another.* ~~ George Eliot

While the social branch of soul health describes the
characters who may play a part in our human drama,
the interpersonal branch relates to the dynamics we develop in our
relationships with them. As noted, many people enter therapy because
their relationships need work. Our interactions with others start to
take form from the second we are born, and they begin with how
we are cared for and taught. This sets the stage, informing us about
our parents' and caregivers' perceptions of the world. In many cases
a healthy dynamic is formed; but in many, the key ingredients are
skewed or missing, leaving us with thoughts, beliefs, and behavior
that may negatively affect relationships we develop later in life.

The way we see people interact during our childhood often
programs our ideas and expectations of later relationships. When
our experiences with others fail to match those expectations we can

have a rude awakening. Although many people recapitulate—or recreate—dynamics similar to those we experienced in our families of origin, whether healthy or not, they often do so unconsciously. We often hear of people "marrying" a parent, or someone with a combination of both parents' characteristics, meaning that they fall into patterns with their partner that are influenced by a dominant or influential parent or parents. They do this because it is a familiar dynamic, not necessarily a healthy or fulfilling one. This dynamic will be discussed further later in this chapter. But first, complete the following questionnaire to help assess the health of your interpersonal relationships.

QUESTIONNAIRE FOR THE INTERPERSONAL BRANCH OF HEALTH

On a scale of 1 to 10, rate the level of your health within each area described. A 10 describes optimal, radiant health, while a 1 describes an almost complete lack of health within the given aspect of the interpersonal branch. Remember, this questionnaire is designed to create a roadmap to overall radiant health. It is not meant to overwhelm you.

Communication

1. _____ I communicate well with the people in my life and they would agree.
2. _____ I communicate my feelings and needs well to those in my life.
3. _____ I am able to talk about difficult things with those in my life.
4. _____ I consider my friends and family to be good communicators.
5. _____ I limit the time I spend with people who don't communicate well.

Boundaries

1. _____ I know what healthy boundaries are.
2. _____ I have good physical and emotional boundaries with people in my life.
3. _____ I respect other people's boundaries.
4. _____ I can say no to others when I need to.
5. _____ I know when a personal boundary has been breached and I actively reestablish it.
6. _____ I avoid people who don't have good boundaries.
7. _____ I feel emotionally and physically safe with the people in my life.

Personal Integrity

1. _____ I know what personal integrity is.
2. _____ I only do things that feel right to me.
3. _____ I work to maintain the integrity of my relationships with others.
4. _____ I maintain my own personal integrity despite what others may say or do.
5. _____ I only spend time with those who respect my personal integrity.

Equality

1. _____ I know what equal partnership means.
2. _____ Friends, family, and my partner see me as an equal and treat me accordingly.
3. _____ I see and treat my friends, family, and partner as equals.
4. _____ My relationships with others are equally life-giving.

Respect

1. _____ My actions show that I respect myself completely.
2. _____ I feel completely respected by those in my life and I respect them completely.
3. _____ I feel respected by the people in my life even though they may not like what I say or do.
4. _____ I respect the people in my life even though I may not like what they say or do.

Unconditionality

1. _____ I know what it means to be unconditional toward myself and others.
2. _____ I unconditionally accept myself.
3. _____ I unconditionally accept my friends, family, and partner.
4. _____ Friends, family, and my partner unconditionally accept me.
5. _____ I see my own and others' judgments as cues to become more unconditional in some way.
6. _____ I can remain unconditional toward others even if they judge, hurt, or offend me.

As you read through the questions, you likely identified relationships in your life that may need adjustment in order to create healthier and more fulfilling interactions. Our yearning for healthier, stronger and/or compassionate interactions is our soul's request for investing in our relationships. We all know when there is discourse between us and others and it is our soul that measures or monitors this discontent.

IDEAL INTERACTIONS

When people care for you and cry for you, they can straighten out your soul. ~~ Langston Hughes

Numerous models exist which instruct us about how to create healthy relationships. But, to me, the six qualities assessed above are the key components necessary for a relationship to serve your optimal interpersonal health. You may have noticed, while completing the questionnaire, that each of the qualities depends on the others—without one quality, it is impossible to have the others. In this way, they are much like the branches of soul health, whose complex qualities are also inter-reliant. When one is out of balance, so are the others. This is why relationships are so challenging. First you must know yourself—know your soul—well enough to know what *you* need in order to remain healthy; then you must bring people into your life who can sustain, rather than diminish, the health of your soul. This is also why relationships are such fertile ground for our soul development; they force us to become both aware and respectful of the voice of our soul. When we don't, our overall soul health is threatened and often compromised.

The six core characteristics of interpersonal soul health are communication, integrity, boundaries, equality, respect and unconditionality. Other key qualities are also necessary to interpersonal branch, but they are all characteristics of the six listed above. For instance, one cannot have honesty in a relationship without having integrity; there is no compassion if there is no respect; and one cannot be accepting without unconditionality. So, although we may describe many qualities we want from our relationships, each is reflected in those listed above. To understand each characteristic further, I offer the explanations below.

COMMUNICATION

Electric communication will never be a substitute for the face of someone who with their soul encourages another person to be brave and true. ~~ Charles Dickens

Probably the most common complaint about relationships relates to communication. Few people really learn to communicate in a conscious manner, let alone to listen with full attention. Even our high school or college speech classes are designed to either instruct or influence others rather than to converse with and understand them. So it is not surprising that few actually know how to have a heart-to-heart talk, let alone one that is soul-to-soul. Even fewer people know how to listen unless they have learned by good example. Conscious communication requires us to engage in purely honest, clear, and direct interactive conversation with others, but from a non-critical, non-judgmental perspective. At the same time, we must avoid defensive reactions in order to hear and understand another's perspective. Effective communication happens only when both parties feel heard and neither goes away feeling dismissed. This is not to say that each has to agree with the other's viewpoint—they just have to hear and understand it. Throughout a conscious conversation, other qualities such as honesty, assertiveness, and acceptance are maintained as well.

However, our soul knows when we are holding back. When we fail to communicate our needs, wishes, or frustrations, we manifest *dis*-ease in other areas of soul health. For example, anxiety and/or depression often emerge from un-communicated feelings and thoughts. Other unhealthy reactions can unknowingly develop as we avoid expressing ourselves. For example, emotional eating habits—a way of filling an emotional void instead of feeding genuine hunger—often develops as a result of "eating" or "swallowing" the words we wish we could or would say. The "pit" in our stomach or "frog" in our throats can also manifest from unsaid words. Multiple physical manifestations of unaddressed emotional issues are possible. Throat problems (chronic coughing, sore throats, laryngitis) and intestinal issues (stomach upset, ulcers, diarrhea, constipation) are not uncommon in those who have difficulty communicating their thoughts and feelings to others. We need to tune in to these muffled voices if we want to understand our truth and honor our soul.

» Do you feel heard by those in your life?

» Do others shut down or change the subject when you are talking about tough situations?

» Are you able to express your full range of emotions?

» Do you find yourself or others in your life voicing only half-truths?

» Is dishonesty a part of your relationships?

BOUNDARIES

My soul is not my own any more. I cannot live like I want to. ~~ Brigitte Bardot

Boundaries indicate a limit or border. In relationships they can easily become blurred. In order to maintain clear boundaries, you must not only know your own limits, but also those of others. Unfortunately, we can lose sight of our boundaries simply by trying to please those around us. Similar to the other elements of relationships, our ideas about boundaries were likely instilled in us during childhood. If those around us did not respect each other's boundaries, including our own, we may have difficulty setting and maintaining boundaries later in life.

Ideas of boundaries can apply to any branch of soul health. Physical boundaries protect your physical needs (safety, security, nutrition, exercise, sleep). Emotional boundaries help you set realistic expectations for your life, assert yourself, avoid taking things personally, guard against manipulation, and appropriately assess your self-worth. Financial boundaries can be protected by setting and maintaining a budget, paying your bills on time, putting money aside for your future, and not lending to others unless your own needs are met. A breach in any or all of these boundaries can disrupt your relationships and damage your overall soul health.

Our gut reactions generally let us know when we have breached a key boundary and whether we need to retreat from something we've done or retract something we've said. These reactions can help to guide us even when our intellect can't. In particular, a sense of regret is a clear indication that we ignored or defied our gut or soul, thus, causing our own suffering as a result of our actions and decisions. Even if the heart or head creates blurred boundaries, our gut reactions, once interpreted correctly, provide the clarity we need to protect our interpersonal soul health.

» Do others accept it when you tell them no?

» Do you feel pressured to do things you don't want to (like eating, drinking, having sex)

» Do you offer to do things when you really don't want to or because you feel you have no choice?

INTEGRITY

The man who is always worrying about whether or not his soul would be damned generally has a soul that isn't worth a damn. ~~ Oliver Wendell Holmes

Many people talk about self-esteem as an important part of healthy relationships. Although I agree, I prefer to talk to clients about integrity instead. Low self-esteem comes from living life—or comparing oneself to others— from the outside in, which causes people to constantly check the world around them to see if they are "okay". They use external measures to determine their worth and to assess whether they are good enough for the world at large. This is tricky, and it often creates an emotional trap since the world around us holds many unhealthy ideas about whom and what we should and shouldn't be. The problem is that these ideas change all the time.

Integrity, however, is living from the inside out, which is more consistent with soul health. In contrast to self-esteem, integrity develops from following what feels right for *you* with respect to your inner truth—your soul—instead of trying to satisfy those around you (which is often impossible anyway). Integrity is "the state of being whole, entire or undiminished", which also defines radiant soul health. When you exercise your integrity, your actions reflect what is right for your soul. This is not to say that you will act without morality or ethics as you serve your innermost needs. It only means that you will honor your soul through your actions, which is the true source of integrity.

Integrity is sometimes hard to maintain in relationships. If one party has low self-esteem, their insecurity may affect the other's ability to maintain their own integrity, especially if the stronger person feels guilty or sorry for the one who is insecure. This may cause the person with intact self-esteem to loosen their personal boundaries and dismiss the voice of their soul out of pity for the other person. This can be incredibly damaging not only for the one feeling guilt, but for the couple as well. Both parties are responsible for his or her self-esteem and integrity. Keeping this clearly in mind will allow each to consciously assess any unhealthy self-perceptions that may exist. Doing so will greatly enhance the health of not only the relationship, but each person's soul.

» Is jealously part of your relationships?

» Does insecurity—yours or others'—inhibit strong bonds in your life?

» Do you need constant reassurance from others in your life or do they need that from you?

» Do you or others in your life have to apologize often?

EQUALITY

The soul that is within me no man can degrade. ~~ Frederick Douglass

If any type of relationship has changed throughout the years, it is the idea of marriage and committed partnership. In earlier times, the breadwinner had more power in the relationship than his or her partner. Most marriages were unequal unions. Today, equality has to do with equal participation in the development and maintenance of relationships. Ideally, neither person feels degraded or less valued in the union. In domestic partnership, this may mean equal sharing of household duties and expenses, and equal responsibility for child care. Decision making is a joint effort, and life's changes are met with open discussion about how to manage any shifts of responsibility. While intimate partnerships require equality, other relationships— friendships, family relationships, work relations, and so on— are all subject to this element of healthy relationships.

In all relationships, equality relates back to whether the dynamic is equally life-affirming for everyone involved. Generally, the give and take nature of any relationship should feel balanced for all, with no lasting resentment or anger stemming from the parties' interactions. For any individual to maintain personal power—a strong sense of self separate from a relationship—all parties involved must actively develop and uphold the equality of the other.

A person firmly in touch with his or her soul sees all others as equals. No factor—not race, gender, culture, income, education, or circumstance sets one soul apart from another. Healthy souls have no need to place limits or deny the equality of others.

» Do you do more for others than they do for you?

» Do you make important decisions only after discussing them with others who will be affected?

» Are you resentful about what others do— or don't— do for you?

» Do you see others as your equals? Do those around you see you as an equal?

RESPECT

Belief consists in accepting the affirmations of the soul; unbelief, in denying them. ~~ George Eliot

If you wish to be to be respected, you must respect yourself first. If you deny your soul, then others will as well. Along with esteem and self-worth, self-respect is built on both action and reverence on behalf of self and others. Without respect, no other qualities of the interpersonal branch of health are possible. To respect others, then, is to uphold their worth, regardless of whether you agree with their ideas, beliefs, or actions. This does not mean that you always have to follow their lead, give in to their whims, or alter your own course to suit them. It only means that you accept their path as their own.

Self-respect is also the strongest form of protection for your soul. It is the acknowledgement that your inner truth or wisdom is worth defending. Without self-respect, you will be more easily manipulated by others, offending the voice of your soul. To achieve radiant soul health, you must not only listen to your inner voice, but also respect and honor its requests. By respecting your soul, you will more easily and fully balance all branches of soul health.

» Do others often interrupt you? When they do, do you speak up or let it go?

» Are your opinions accepted by others?

» Do you assert yourself when necessary?

» Do you engage in unhealthy behaviors, such as emotional eating, after you feel you've been disrespected?

UNCONDITIONALITY

Compassion is the antitoxin of the soul. Where there is compassion even the most poisonous impulses remain relatively harmless. ~~ Eric Hoffer

We have all known people who placed conditions on us for their attention, affection or approval. In doing so, they limit our ability to thrive and diminish our ability to be ourselves. They violate all other qualities of healthy interpersonal relations.

Parenting coach and writer Scott Noelle describes unconditionality as a state of mind in which you are willing to allow well-being into your experiences and others'. He notes that by adopting an unconditional approach to life you will experience more freedom, joy, and appreciation. How, then, do we get others to do the same? This is the greatest challenge in interpersonal relations.

Everyone wants to be freely understood and openly accepted, but very few people are. Instead, most of us are constantly challenged to conform to the ideas of others, whether those of our families, culture, religions, society, or workplace. We are ingrained with the limits of our immediate experience and often fail to challenge these despite the declining health of our soul. A commitment to soul health means adopting an unconditional approach to your own life as well as that of others.

As Helen Keller said, "Character cannot be developed in ease and quiet. Only through experience of trial and suffering can the soul be strengthened, ambition inspired, and success achieved." Just think how much easier it would be to honor our soul if we all achieved more unconditionality for ourselves and toward others.

» Do you feel judged by others?

» Do you hold back in what you say or do to appease another person's beliefs or ideas?

» How often do you judge yourself?

» Are you unconditional toward *you*?

REPEAT PERFORMANCES

Have you noticed that how you react in one relationship is also how you tend to react in others? Do you feel pressured, harried, or made to feel guilty by more than one person in your life? Whether with friends, family, coworkers, neighbors, or other peripheral relationships, we tend to repeat certain interpersonal dynamics in many or all of our connections.

These repeat performances are indications or red flags that our interpersonal health needs work—that we need to evolve beyond the dynamic we seem to be repeating. If you continually find yourself getting hurt, angry, or frustrated with others, it's time to take a look at your behavior to identify the faulty pattern. Chances are, the dynamic was unconsciously ingrained in you at an early age but no longer works for the sake of your soul. As we consciously choose to become healthier, evolution beyond our old patterns is essential. Otherwise we continue to experience distressing—and even disturbing—replications of previous interaction. As Albert Einstein said "Insanity is doing the same thing over and over again but expecting different results." Sometimes this means changing what we do or how we react, and in some cases it means eliminating a relationship altogether. Anything that you experience repeatedly is likely to be a major life lesson waiting to be identified as something to evolve beyond. We all repeat the same mistakes because we are creatures of habit. But, as the most conscious creatures on earth, we are also the most capable of changing our unhealthy dynamics.

The Interpersonal branch of soul health clearly affects all others. Without conscious awareness of the dynamics of our relationships we will inhibit not only our soul health, but also our evolution. There is a reason fish evolved beyond the sea, and there are reasons why we, as humans, are to evolve beyond our old ways of living as well.

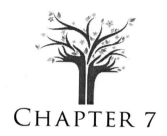

CHAPTER 7

INTELLECTUAL/ OCCUPATIONAL HEALTH: CONSCIOUS COGNITIONS

The soul becomes dyed by the color of its thoughts. ~~ Marcus Aurelius

The human species is known for its brain. It is the central processing unit that most defines us as human, and yet it eludes its researchers' full understanding. Scientists remain baffled by not only its inherent capabilities, but also by its power of adaptation. Although some species exhibit certain levels of conscious thought, we hold the bar for advanced cognitive processing.

Our ability to think is essential in the work force. According to the American Time Use Survey, U.S. citizens spend more time working (8.6 hours) than they do sleeping (7.6 hours). Work occupies nearly 60 percent of our waking hours, though many spend much longer hours at their jobs. Clearly, if one is unsatisfied, overwhelmed, or simply bored with their work, their soul health will inevitably suffer.

Life presents many other opportunities to think, solve problems, and reflect on ideas, actions, and beliefs. Students, retired people, stay-at-home parents, avid readers, volunteers, and those who explore creative or artistic talents also pursue mentally stimulating activities to enhance soul health.

Our intellectual and occupational health includes our pursuit of creating and maintaining an intellectually stimulating life— it is our human quest for knowledge and skill. Although for many this does, in fact, include a job or career, this branch of health also describes our ability to develop or maintain a strong cognitive capacity. Our intellectual health depends on mental stimulation, a curiosity and drive to learn, a willingness and ability to engage in effective and conscious thought processing, intellectual clarity and adaptability, the insight necessary to integrate our perceptions of the world, the assimilation of new concepts, exercise and maintenance of memory, and the ability to reason between right and wrong. Simply put, whether we are mentally over-stimulated or bored to tears, our level of intellectual and health can affect our overall experience of soul health.

What do you do to enhance your cognitive abilities? What keeps you sharp? What challenges your brain? What dulls it? When are you the most curious or interested in something? When are you the most bored? What helps you to think clearly? And what serves to distract you? How does creativity affect your life?

While knowledge is the ultimate human quest, we must also remember that knowledge also allows our souls to evolve. As we expand our minds— learn and grow as human beings—, our souls expand as well. This is especially true within the context of consciousness—and even more so when we become "radical" in its pursuit. Those who become increasingly conscious about how they are living their lives open themselves to the greatest opportunities for evolution. This 3-D method of living— the ability to recognize a depth of meaning beyond what is right in front of you — allows the human condition to become our classroom— we learn how best we can learn! Thus, our soul's quest for growth depends greatly on how we consciously use our brains to evolve.

CEREBRAL STIMULATION

And what, Socrates, is the food of the soul? Surely, I
said, knowledge is the food of the soul. ~~ Plato

Some people are more conscious than others in their quest for intellectual health. Our pursuit of education is likely the strongest indicator of this quest. From a very early age, we become curious about the world. We explore, we learn, we succeed, we fail— all in the pursuit of mental stimulation. As with all things, people have varying degrees of interest in this pursuit. Many have a hunger for learning; others are satisfied with maintaining what they have; while others resist all methods of learning regardless of how they are presented. Those who crave knowledge seek it in a variety if ways—formally, through advanced education, or through exploring mental activities on their own .

Knowledge is the one thing that can never be taken away; all else can. English writer, G.K. Chesterton stated that "Education is simply the soul of a society as it passes from one generation to another." But whether we choose to be educated through formal means or by life itself, expanding our knowledge and skills can keep us healthier and more satisfied than those who do not choose to enhance their intellectual health. Research on life satisfaction clearly reinforces this notion.

But education itself is only part of the story. Most important to intellectual health are factors inherent to the individual, but not necessarily trainable through formal education.

The first half of the Intellectual/Occupational Health Quiz pertains to mental stimulation, curiosity/passion and thought processes—all of which affect our general intellectual health. The remaining half relates more to people who are in the workforce and assesses their sense of control, ability to manage responsibilities, and their openness to change. These focus on these qualities reflects the impact of the current employment culture, since all are constructs that can affect our intellectual/occupational health. Complete the quiz now to understand more about this branch of your soul health.

Questionnaire for the Intellectual/ Occupational Branch of Health

On a scale of 1 to 10, rate the level of your health within each area described. A 10 describes optimal, radiant health, while a 1 describes an almost complete lack of health within the given aspect of the intellectual/ occupation branch. Remember, this questionnaire is designed to create a roadmap to overall radiant health. It is not meant to overwhelm you.

Mental Stimulation
1. ____ I feel mentally challenged by the activities in my work and home life.
2. ____ My life is mentally stimulating and interesting.
3. ____ Generally, I do not feel bored.
4. ____ I actively use my creativity in my life.
5. ____ I engage in activities that keep my thoughts and memory sharp.

Curiosity and Passion
1. ____ I am excited about my life.
2. ____ I am naturally curious about how things work.
3. ____ I actively pursue things I'm passionate about.
4. ____ I am constantly trying to learn new things.
5. ____ I feel satisfied with the activities in my life.
6. ____ I am personally invested in everything I do

Thought Processes
1. ____ I easily maintain my train of thought.
2. ____ I am a good problem solver.
3. ____ My memory is sharp.
4. ____ Generally, I can remember what I have recently read.
5. ____ I have clear, un-muddled thoughts.
6. ____ I make decisions easily.

Sense of Control
1. ____ I have a sense of control in intellectual tasks.
2. ____ I have control in my work environment.
3. ____ I can negotiate with others in my work environment to meet mutual needs.
4. ____ Changes at work are discussed openly.
5. ____ People in my work environment value my opinion.

Responsibilities
1. ____ My daily responsibilities are reasonable.
2. ____ I feel good about what I accomplish.
3. ____ I can easily accomplish my responsibilities.
4. ____ I rarely feel overwhelmed.

Openness to Change
1. ____ I am open to change.
2. ____ I adapt well to change.
3. ____ I don't take changes made by others personally.
4. ____ I see change as a new challenge.
5. ____ I believe that periodic change can benefit me in some way.

MENTAL STIMULATION

Whatever feeds our brain also feeds our soul. Mental stimulation can become intoxicating, leaving us wanting more. But when we feed our minds with toxic or unhealthy ideas, we can threaten— and even damage— both our intellectual health as well as the health of our soul. Rarely does a person feel mentally stimulated by a task, job, or subject that they hate. In fact, in a recent online survey, 86 percent of workers responded that they would choose a new job based on mental stimulation, and 39 percent would choose a career path that offered a new job opportunity over a a job with a higher salary. So, although money can be motivator, it is not everything to everyone.

Without mental stimulation we would not evolve. Our soul would be bored and under-nourished. And because we must work in tandem with our soul to evolve, what prompts us to use our brains in healthy ways also stimulates and satisfies our soul.

» Do you like your work and/or feel adequately stimulated by your life?

» Does your work, or your life, leave you wanting more?

» Are you happy to arrive at work?

» Does your life feel meaningful to you— like you are making a difference in some way?

CURIOSITY/PASSION

Curiosity is the desire to learn and to *know*. Passion is having boundless enthusiasm or a strong liking for something. Both are driving forces in attaining intellectual/occupational health.

Although research on curiosity and cognition is not extensive, it does indicate that the more curious employee, the more likely to adjust to job-related changes, to new careers, to report higher job satisfaction, to perform at a higher level, and to achieve greater and faster job-related learning. However, when the research assesses passion, the results are mixed. Some authors assert that a passion for work increases job satisfaction, while others claim it can actually diminish satisfaction if workplace obstacles make it hard to fulfill this passion.

No one could deny, however, that having a vested interest in your work actually helps your overall life satisfaction. In fact, it is necessary to soul health. A bored or passionless soul does not thrive. Instead, it becomes stagnant and dark. In contrast, an endless curiosity or hunger for knowledge and growth lights up both the mind and soul.

» Do you have a constant hunger to learn more?

» Does your work reflect your intellectual passions?

» Do you invest in the time it takes to learn new things?

THOUGHT PROCESSING

The ability to focus our thoughts plays a big part in every aspect of our everyday lives, but especially in our work satisfaction. Many factors can undermine our ability to effectively process our thoughts, and thereby damage soul health as well. These include stress, depression, anxiety, sleeplessness, a sense of overwhelm, distractibility, medical illness or structural changes in the brain (memory loss or altered functioning), as well as chemical or other dependency (addictions other than drugs or alcohol). However, this also works two ways—personal issues can interfere with your ability to focus on work or your work life can disrupt your attention to life outside of work, especially if you are suffering from burnout, low job satisfaction, high levels of stress, or heavy pressure to produce.

When our thought processes become blurred, scattered or broken, they can create a similar effect on our soul.

» Do you find yourself daydreaming at work?

» Do your thoughts often feel scrambled and disorganized?

» Are you making mistakes because you have too much to think about?

» Are you forgetting what you were going to do next?

WORK ENVIRONMENT

*My mouth is full of decayed teeth and my soul
of decayed ambitions.* ~~ James Joyce

It is one thing to feel motivated and stimulated by a job or career and another thing to find a work environment in which you can truly thrive. Whether you are working at a job or not, your intellectual health depends on how you perceive your current situation. Your sense of control, level of responsibility, and openness to change can all be affected by your work environment, and in turn affect how satisfied you are with your work life and, thus, your life in general.

SENSE OF CONTROL

Job stress is often a function of how much control an employee has at work. Many studies indicate that job satisfaction and productivity decrease, and absenteeism increases, when workers have little control over their working conditions, decisions made, or hours that they work. As modern work environment shift, people have less and less control over job stability, attainment of personal goals, and pursuit of their career-related passions. Experts say that workers will undergo between five and seven career changes in their lifetime, with several job changes for each. In tough economic times, employees may shift careers more to ensure gainful employment than to fulfill their true interests, let alone their souls.

> » Do you have the kinds of control you need in order to thrive in your job?

> » Do you avoid conflict at work simply to keep your job?

> » Do you fear being handed a pink slip every time you go to work?

> » When was the last time you felt you had the control you need in order to thrive?

RESPONSIBILITIES

What I hear most from clients about their work lives are: 1) that they have too much to do and 2) that they aren't doing the work they were hired to do. In neither case do they feel fulfilled. In many cases, employees don't feel sufficiently trained to perform well at their jobs, and yet they feel their managers or supervisors still don't provide the support they need. Many simply lose their jobs if they can't or won't do what is required to complete assigned tasks.

But an overworked human eventually leads to an overworked soul. Because our soul thrives on new opportunities for growth, an experience that leaves a person burned out can do the same to that person's soul.

> » Are you able to comfortably manage your responsibilities at work?

» Are you doing more than you were hired to do?

» Does your skill set match your responsibilities?

OPENNESS TO CHANGE

Change is the most constant variable in the world of work. One cannot work for someone else and not be expected to change. And even self-employed people must adjust to the the economy, to supply and demand, and to governing bodies that create the policies and rules for professional practice. Those who resist change will have the most difficult time adjusting to new or different responsibilities, schedules, and coworkers. However, those who see change as a challenge or a new opportunity will more likely welcome it.

Ironically, it is often change that dislodges our soul from a sense that we are stuck— in a routine, in a dead-end job or career, and in work that no longer offers a challenge. When we embrace change as necessary to growth, we move through it more easily, smoothly, and quickly.

» How do you approach change?

» How do you usually make transitions to new responsibilities?

» How do you feel in the course of changes?

As you read about the intellectual branch of soul health, you are likely gaining a better understanding of its impact on overall well-being. A fulfilling intellectual/occupational life often sets the stage for the rest of life satisfaction. Given that we spend over 1/3 of our lives at work, it goes without saying that our fulfillment of this branch inevitably influences our soul health.

CONSCIOUS CALLINGS

All things must come to the soul from its roots, from where it is planted. ~~ Saint Teresa of Avila

One cannot talk about intellectual health and not mention the idea of hearing a "call". Plato saw thinking as the *talking of the soul itself*. Certainly we need our brains to translate what the soul wants to convey, but the soul also needs the brain to identify and process its truth. Aligning our human condition—most directly represented through our perceptions of it—, with our soul or spirit condition—, the awareness and use of our inner wisdom—, is what shows us our calling. Only when we integrate with both does our calling in life emerge.

Many feel spontaneously "called" to their life's work while others yearn to hear their own calling. Author Mary Jaksch describes a calling as *an abiding passion that shapes your life.* She notes that life becomes more meaningful once you align with your passion, since this sets the stage for your life's mission. Although a calling can be instrumental in guiding life's path, very few actually listen for, hear, and find it. As long as a person feels intellectually fulfilled in their life or their work, their soul can find contentment without a calling. Most people don't even need the ideal job or career to do so, just the conscious effort to satisfy their intellectual needs.

Countless situations and circumstances affect intellectual/occupational fulfillment and thus, our soul health: burnout, job loss—your own or those around you—, adjusting to retirement or re-entering the workforce when financially necessary, shifts in interests, abilities, or priorities and far too many more to address here. But the fact remains that how we develop and engage our brain is directly connected to the satisfaction of our soul, and if our intellect is left unfulfilled, our soul health will suffer.

Take some time to re-examine the graphic of the Soul Health Model in chapter two so that you can refresh your sense of the many ways in which the branches of health impact one another in your own life. By now you will see how their interactions may be shaping you own life and health. The ability to think your way through the model is essential identifying difficulties that can undermine your soul's health and evolution. The point of reviewing the model is not to overwhelm you; rather, it is simply to expand your awareness—your consciousness—about the intricacies and interactions of the branches on the health of your soul.

CHAPTER 8

ENVIRONMENTAL HEALTH:
INSIDE AWARENESS OF THE OUTSIDE WORLD

*Humans and nature belong together, in their created glory, in
their great tragedy, and in their salvation.* ~~ Paul Tillich

Theologian, Paul Tillich wrote the epitaph quoted above as he
reflected on his relationship with environment late in his life.
Our relationship with the world around us— immediate, global, and
universal— is much like the relationships we have with our self and
others. Either we value and take care of it or we don't. This connection
mirrors how we see and treat ourselves and others and ultimately
reflects our connection with our soul.

Ancient cultures were intimately involved with their external
environment. They not only depended on it directly and immediately
for their survival, but also relied greatly on their connection to the
very soul of the earth—their most valued guide— for their evolution.
They did not separate themselves from their planetary host; instead
they embraced the union, paying homage with every action and
through every breath. What modern cultures often see as simply the

workings of the world with little direct connection to human lives, the ancients saw and experienced as a deeper and richer bond. They interacted with their immediate environment, the planet on which they lived, and the expanded universe as they would with another person—another soul. Most of us today have little understanding of the connection between our external environment and our innermost ally. The less connected we are with our environment, the less connected we are to our soul.

The environmental branch of soul health reflects not only our relationship with our immediate, global, and universal surroundings, but with our internal world—our soul. Often, our outside environment reflects how we feel inside. If we feel scattered and messy on the inside, we are generally scattered and messy on the outside as well. If we have an obsessive disposition, we will likely be obsessive about our environment. If we don't really care about the world around us, we don't generally invest in our inner world either. Of course there are exceptions, but in most cases, our soul is a mirror of how we see and maintain the world around us.

This branch also pertains to safety, security and overall maintenance of our external environment— how well ordered, clean and functional we keep it. This represents the *science* aspect of our basic survival which has to do with whether we create an environment that is conducive to soul health. At the same time, the emotional environment around us— for example, the sense of tension or ease— often dictates how we *feel* in a particular physical space, which in turn can have an impact on our soul. Thus, we must actively preserve and promote both our inner world and outside world in order for the sake of our soul's evolution.

ENVIRONMENTAL HEALTH

Pleasure is nature's test, her sign of approval. When man is happy, he is in harmony with himself and his environment. ~~ Oscar Wilde

According to the World Health Organization (WHO), environmental health pertains to all physical, chemical, and biological factors external to a person that impact health. The WHO's main mission is to educate society to create a health-supportive environment by raising people's awareness about their everyday choices and behavior.

The Soul Health Model takes the environmental branch of health further. Not only is it important for people to understand how their behavior either promotes or undermines a health-supportive environment, it is also imperative to create an environment conducive to the soul's evolution. When we think about environmental health, we tend to focus on factors that support our basic needs— the *science* aspect of our surroundings. Equally important, though, is an awareness of what we need to truly feed our soul— the *art* aspect of creating this environment. For some, this may mean paying attention to the aesthetic qualities around them, while for others it might mean surrounding themselves with objects that instill a sense of peace or inspiration. Developing the *art* of creating a soulful environment simply means that you have an awareness of what you need that resonates deeply within your soul. Achieving a balance between the *science*- and *art*-based elements of the environmental branch allows us to thrive— and allows our soul to evolve.

The following questionnaire will help you assess your environmental branch of health. As you will see, it is more than the beauty of our surroundings that creates a healthy environment.

QUESTIONNAIRE FOR THE ENVIRONMENTAL BRANCH OF HEALTH

On a scale of 1 to 10, rate the level of your health within each area described. A 10 describes optimal, radiant health, while a 1 describes an almost complete lack of health within the given aspect of the environmental branch. Remember, this questionnaire is designed to create a roadmap to overall radiant health. It is not meant to overwhelm you.

Healthy Hearth
1. ____ I live in clean, safe, and healthy surroundings.
2. ____ I like where I live (my neighborhood, state, country, and climate).
3. ____ I live and work in clutter-free environments.
4. ____ I take care of my personal environment.
5. ____ I practice regular home maintenance and safety measures (change filters, check for leaks, etc.).
6. ____ My home provides good shelter (is insulated, free of drafts, leaks, etc.).
7. ____ I work to reduce pollution in my environment (air, chemical, noise, etc.).

Aesthetics
1. ____ My personal surroundings fit who I am.
2. ____ My work surroundings fit who I am.
3. ____ I take pleasure in what I place in my surroundings.
4. ____ I know what I need around me to feel safe, comfortable, and fulfilled.
5. ____ I actively rid myself of things that don't fit my preferences.
6. ____ I look forward to spending time in my surroundings.

Ecological Impact
1. ____ I understand that how I choose to live affects the environment in which I live.
2. ____ I do not waste food, water, energy, or fuel.
3. ____ I buy and keep only what I need.
4. ____ I only purchase 'eco-friendly' products (appliances, cleaning products, compostable packaging, etc.).
5. ____ I am conscious of minimizing my impact on the environment.
6. ____ I do not litter and always clean up after myself and those I'm responsible for (family, pets. etc.).
7. ____ I avoid using toxic and/or harmful chemicals (cleaning products, pesticides, herbicides, etc.).

Sacred Surroundings
1. ____ I feel connected with the earth.
2. ____ I feel connected with my personal environment.
3. ____ I actively work to make my environment peaceful and calming.
4. ____ My surroundings reflect my core beliefs.
5. ____ I know when I need to reconnect with the earth and with my personal surroundings.
6. ____ I spend time outside to connect with the earth.

Cultural and Emotional Environment
1. ____ I live in a place that fits my cultural beliefs and values.
2. ____ I work in an environment that fits my cultural beliefs and values.
3. ____ My personal environment is calm and without tension.
4. ____ My work environment is calm and free of tension.
5. ____ I live in a trusting environment.
6. ____ I work in a trusting environment.
7. ____ I feel accepted at home and at work.
8. ____ I feel emotionally safe in my environment.

As you can see by completing the questionnaire, the environmental branch of health goes far beyond the air we breathe and the land on which we walk. In order to enjoy soul health, we must be conscious of more than satisfying our most basic needs. We need to assess how well we fit into different aspects of our environment (home, work, the part of the country or world in which we reside, what helps us to feel grounded or at home), and what we need in order for our souls to grow. We must know not only what helps us to feel safe and secure, but also whether we need a rural or urban environment, whether we prefer the ocean, mountains, prairie or desert, which kind of climate we thrive in—or are repelled by—, what types of people we enjoy spending time with (cultural backgrounds, beliefs, personalities, interests), what impact we have on the natural environment, and where we need to spend time in order to grow spiritually. Our consciousness about these needs and our ability to fulfill them is important if we are to find and develop an environment that supports not only the health of our bodies, but also the health of our souls.

Consider the following aspects of environmental health more carefully in assessing how "soul supportive" your environment is.

HEALTHY HEARTH

Every spirit builds itself a house, and beyond its house, a world, and beyond its world, a heaven. Know then that world exists for you." ~~ Ralph Waldo Emerson

The most common ideas people have about environmental health encompass what I call the "healthy hearth". These include access to food and water, shelter, safety, a comfortable climate, minimal exposure to pollutants, cleanliness, order (lack of clutter), and an ongoing pride of ownership that comes from taking care of one's personal environment and belongings. Together, these qualities fulfill basic needs and represent the *science* aspects of our environment we need in order to survive and even thrive.

Many of us take for granted the luxury of a warm, dry environment in which we feel safe and secure. In the most basic terms, all we need is a roof over our heads, a place to stay warm and dry, and enough food and water to eat and drink to stay alive. But in our world today, a healthy hearth seems to require much more. As the world has evolved, technology, especially, has greatly improved more than just our ability to meet our basic needs. We no longer need to rely only on immediate resources to survive; we now expect our environments to help us thrive. Accessibility of goods and convenience of services also reflect our modern environment. All of these factors directly impact our general well-being and soul health.

» How well are your most basic needs met?

» Do you feel pride of ownership toward your living space and for your belongings?

» Are you personally invested in maintaining your immediate surroundings?

» Do you feel healthy in your environment? What could you do to feel more so?

AESTHETICS

Everybody needs beauty as well as bread, places to lay in and pray in, where nature may heal and give strength to body and soul. ~~ John Muir

Although we all require our basic needs to be met—the *science* of survival—, it is often the *art* of creating an aesthetic environment that feeds our souls most. This is why most civilizations have created sculptures, monuments, architecture, artwork, weaponry, ornate styles of dress, ornamental jewelry, other elaborate accessories, and intricate spiritual and religious symbols — which often reflect stages of their own evolution. Egyptian, Mayan, Aztec, Incan, Aborigine, African, Native Americans and many other cultures developed meaningful symbols which reflected their connection between the environment, their self, and their soul. Of course, whatever we need in our immediate surroundings in order to feel whole depends on individual tastes, preferences, and beliefs, but many people give little thought to why they are so drawn to particular objects, colors, textures, scents, sounds, or forms. Although materialism in our culture today often indicates our place in society, few of the items we keep truly feed our souls; they simply take up space.

Although our basic needs remain fairly standard for survival, our individual needs for aesthetic expression—the manner in which we "decorate" our environment— tend to differ widely. What is most important to our soul's health is whether the setting in which we find ourselves suits or expresses who we are at the deepest level. For instance, if you are a city person you likely will not find a rural environment satisfying, and vice versa. Some people need to see open green space or deep woods when they look around them, others prefer buildings, cars, and subways. Nothing in a person's environment can restrict soul health as long as those settings fit their survival and innermost aesthetic needs.

I, for one, enjoy visiting large cities occasionally but prefer to live in a quiet, semi-rural environment. I literally *need* trees around me in order to feel at home, and I choose to live on a densely wooded site in order to bring nature right up to my doorstep. When I go on vacation, I generally choose places even deeper into nature—the less-travelled roads within national parks and natural monuments, as well as the back roads I choose in order to get there. I feel more fully aligned with my soul when immersed in a natural environment, though others may not get the same feeling. Many feel more comfortable in a bustling city, full of the sights, sounds and smells of the urban setting.

As mentioned above, the aesthetic aspect of the environmental branch of health includes how we choose to enhance our immediate environment. Some feel more satisfied amid simple, minimalistic styles, while others feel their growth is most supported by owning more elaborately detailed items (artwork, sculptures, and so on). Some need nature motifs; others modern or abstract art. Some need the quiet sounds of nature; others require the sounds of cars, crowds, and other city noises to feel most at ease. Some prefer soft earth tones to primary bold colors. Some may enjoy living in small spaces, while others are more drawn to large, expansive dwellings and plenty of land. What creates a health-supportive environment depends on beholder's soul. The challenge is to *know* your soul enough to understand what will create this kind of environment for you. This may begin at home, where you have the most control, but you can also make soul-based choices in your work setting, your mode of transportation, and all other aspects of your environment. It is all part of the *art* of living.

» Is your environment health-supportive? What do you need more— or less of— to make them so?

» Do you feel at home where you live and work? What small changes can help you to feel more so?

» What colors, textures, sounds, and smells do you need for your environment to be conducive to both your contentment and your ability to evolve?

ECOLOGICAL IMPACT

*Forests, lakes, and rivers, clouds and winds, stars and
flowers, stupendous glaciers and crystal snowflakes—every
form of animate or inanimate existence leaves its impress
upon the soul of man.* ~~ Orison Swett Marden

However slowly, we seem to be returning to a better relationship with our planet as we hear the warning signs about global warming, scarcity of natural resources, and the negative impact we are creating on earth. Nearly everywhere you look there are signs that we are reawakening to the interconnectedness with nature. Recycling programs, organic gardening, a focus on sustainable living, new forms of eco-friendly structures— both private and corporate—, exploration of cleaner forms of energy, and more efforts urge us to become more conscious of our impact on the earth. It is interesting that these recent developments seem novel, given that our ancestors lived everyday with that awareness, understanding that the circle of life is precious.

Ironically, what we take most for granted is everything that meets our basic needs. If these elements disappeared, we would not survive. Thus, the environmental branch of soul health emphasizes not only stewardship of the earth on which we live, but also our urgent need to maintain a healthy environment for our souls' growth.

There are many ways to become more conscious of your impact on the earth's ecology. A good place to start is to measure the size of the footprint that you leave based on your use of natural resources. You can visit www.carbonfootprint.com to calculate your impact according to the home products you use, the kind of car you drive, how much you travel by car and other means, and many other factors. Simple awareness of your relationship with the world and how you use its resources will help reduce your daily impact.

» Are you mindful of the amount of trash and garbage you generate?

» Do you throw away food often?

» Do you use more plastic than you need to?

» Are you aware of the environmental impact of household cleaners, paint, solvents, and potentially harmful products?

SACRED SURROUNDINGS

To me, it seems a dreadful indignity to have a soul controlled by geography. ~~ George Santayana

Although most ancient cultures created sites sacred to their beliefs—monuments, memorials, ceremonial altars, houses of worship—, not everyone needs formal places in which to feel at peace or to engage with spirit. In fact, it is the *intention* with which we create or maintain our surroundings that makes these places sacred. We can find sacred space simply by choosing or creating an environment in which we feel at peace. Some people may surround themselves with religious or spiritual artifacts and symbols, while others might feel more at peace with the sights and sounds of nature. Whatever connects us most to our own inner wisdom—our soul—is sacred. Thus, a sacred surrounding supports the evolution of our soul.

Certainly magnificent sites around the world inspire the soul to expand. The Pyramids of Egypt, the Taj Mahal of India, the Mayan ruins of Mexico and mystical structures such as Peru's Machu Picchu draw visitors from around the world, many in search of spiritual experiences. However, our personal surroundings can become sacred through our intentions. We can light candles to help us relax and recharge. We can bring nature into the house through flowers and plants, play music to flush out stresses of the day and reconnect with our calmed nature, and prepare food to celebrate our daily existence. Items we choose for everyday rituals are often taken for granted until we place an intention upon them. This is a more conscious means of creating a sacred surrounding. Because we are creatures of habit, our routines—once made intentional—, can create the path to sacred living for our soul's enrichment and growth.

» What do you need around you to feel connected to your soul? To hear your inner wisdom?

» What kind of environment is most conducive to your soul's growth?

» Are your core beliefs reflected in your immediate surroundings?

» What daily routines or rituals do you engage in that could become more sacred if you set intentions for it?

CULTURAL AND "EMOTIONAL" ENVIRONMENT

It is a common habit to blame life upon the environment.
Environment modifies life but does not govern life. The soul
is stronger than its surroundings. ~~ William James

William James' quote shows us that our environment doesn't define us, but it does influence us, particularly if it is not suited to our soul's needs and health. For the sake of our soul health, we must become more aware of how well our environment affirms us and helps our soul to grow. This is true of our immediate surroundings and our broader needs of culture, our lifestyle, and the values by which we live. Because each soul differs in its environmental needs, each of us must consciously assess how our surroundings reflect who we are and whether we can thrive in them. Take, for example, a move to a different part of the country, or another country altogether. Each region or country has its own set of characteristics that may or not match our own soul. Our preferences for climate, country- or city-living, proximity to mountains or the sea, and many other factors all influence whether our souls can thrive. Just because we move to another part of a state or country does not mean our new location will offer the same perspectives on everyday life; in fact, it mostly likely will not. Without this advance awareness, soul health can suffer greatly if we attempt to blend into the culture of a new region despite its ill fit for our soul.

In the United States, endless factors influence the cultural impact of our environment. These include everyday beliefs, traditions, moral values, laws and unwritten rules of behavior, languages spoken, religious observances, customs (including religious ideas about marriage and family), acceptance of gender roles, dietary practices, artistic, intellectual and leisure-time pursuits, ethnic diversity and related customs and beliefs, conceptualization of family, as well as ideas about forms of dress, social mores and overall interpersonal etiquette. All of these subtle—and not so subtle—differences may influence our contentment and thus our environmental soul health.

In other words, we must truly know our soul in order to decipher its complex needs regarding our environmental branch of health. This awareness plays an important role in guiding our soul's evolution. Some value cultural diversity as an opening for growth, while others need a culture they can more readily identify with. Some are hungry to expand their views beyond what is familiar to them; others are content with what they have always known. Neither approach is wrong as long as it fits for our soul at the time.

As a psychologist, I am forever aware of the "emotional" environment in which we work and live. This may be the most influential quality of our environmental health. If our work, home, community or even global environments raise unsettling emotions, these will have a detrimental effect on us. Corporate culture, family tension, environmental disaster, tragic events, and any other emotional element of an environment can drastically alter our sense of comfort or safety. Everyone senses tension or other emotions that can significantly affect their overall ability to function. By creating an emotionally healthy environment we can secure and promote our soul health.

> » Does your cultural environment in which you live reflect who you are? How has this influenced you?

> » Does the culture in which you live help you grow?

> » What sort of emotional environment would be most conducive to your soul's health? (Both work and home.)

NATURAL HISTORY

But ask the animals, and they will teach you; the birds of the air, and they will tell you; ask the plants of the earth, and they will teach you; and the fish of the sea will declare to you. ~~ Job 12:7-8

From the beginning, humans have depended on the earth for their survival. Shelter, safety, security, nourishment, and all other basic needs were provided from the maternal nurturance of our planet, Mother Earth. As humans have grown up, though, we have become less connected to and dependent on our planet and have reached what seems to be an adolescent separation from our primary caregiver. We do depend on the earth, but we try every way possible to deny our dependency. Numerous authors mourn the loss of this relationship and urge humanity to return to the earthly nest by coming to know the soul of the planet once more.

In his book *Nature and the Human Soul*, Bill Plotkin examines how the human race has become as fragmented as the world itself. He writes, "As your ultimate place, your soul is both yours and the world's", and "The human soul, like any soul, cannot be separated from nature." He goes on to say that, "All other creatures seem to take their ultimate place instinctively, unselfconsciously, and without struggle", and "Everything in the universe seems to have been brilliantly designed to take just the place that it does." Plotkin sees humanity as the one exception to this rule, and expresses sadness about our lack of connection with nature.

Just as we no longer directly depend on the earth as we once had in the past, we also no longer turn to it for guidance. All ancient cultures held strong ties to earthly influences. Early hieroglyphics, stone carvings, and cave paintings all reflect the strong influence of fire, wind, water, and animals. Ancient architecture and mystical structures such as Mayan temples, English stone circles, the sculptures on Easter Island, the Nazca Lines of Peru, and others illustrate the early use of astronomy. Any inquiry to early cultures readily reveals their connection with environment. The oldest continuous human culture on this planet is the Australian aboriginal population, which dates back over sixty thousand years. The hallmark of this culture is the belief in humanity's oneness with nature— its interconnectedness with everything—with rocks, canyons, rivers, waterfalls, wind, and all living things, as well as with the stars, moon, sun, and sky itself. Out of this deep reverence for the world around them, they live in unquestionable harmony with the land and everything that lives upon it.

More recent belief systems and healing practices also emphasize a connection with the earth. Chinese medicine is based on the four elements (earth, fire, water, and wind). Native American beliefs give power to the four cardinal directions (north, south, east and west) and attribute symbolic meaning to all living creatures. South American Incan and Mayan cultures built their civilizations around celestial events such as equinoxes and solstices and emphasized Mother Earth and all living creatures as key symbols throughout their existence.

Even the Bible often mentions the important role of nature in the formation of the religious world. Floods, wind, fire, plants, animals, and references to the earth and ground itself abound to illustrate a relationship to God. Author Steven Chase *(Nature as a Spiritual Practice)* explores scripture as a means to reconnect with nature as part of worship and a guide to understanding the world. He emphasizes that nothing is without divine influence or teaching. And most churches, regardless of denomination, continue to use symbols of earthly elements in their religious rituals: incense as earth and wind; baptisms in holy water; fire and the flames of candles as representing the light of God. "Ashes to ashes and dust to dust" illustrates our return to the earth, revered as a deity in and of itself.

It is undeniable that humans would not exist without the planet on which we live. As noted in the Bible verse, Isaiah 24, 4-5: "The earth dries up and withers, the world languishes and withers; the heavens languish together with the earth." We have a symbiotic relationship with the earth: it affects us and we affect it. Either way you look at it, our relationship with our environment and our planet is a reflection on the relationship we hold with our selves—and, more directly, our soul.

» What does the earth mean to you?

» How often do you stop to notice the world around you—the sights, sounds, smells and textures?

» How does your environment—both physical and emotional—impact your overall soul health?

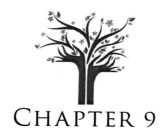

Chapter 9

Financial Health:
A Shift to Sacred Finance

*Suppose you could gain everything in the whole world,
and lost your soul. Was it worth it?* ~~Billy Graham

I n modern society, financial matters threaten our humanity more immediately than many, if not all, of the other aspects of our lives, not only because we need money to live, but because we have placed even greater importance on it than that. Money defines us through what we own, where we live, the clothes we wear, the company we keep, and, especially, the power we might have. We often put more passion into owning things than in tending to our bodies or souls. While our body is the barometer for our physical health, we often see our wallet as the measure of our place in society which too often seems more important than any other aspect of our well-being.

This chapter explores the impacts that our perceptions of money and wealth have on our ability to create balance—or whole health—in our lives. Although our resources are integral to a healthy existence, our perceptions about money can greatly influence the actions, decisions, and outcomes that affect our ability to live radiantly.

Though people might say that our soul has nothing to do with this process, when our ideas about money create stress, greed, insecurity, or other imbalances in life, only the truth of our soul can lead us to peace. Yes, in our society it takes money to survive; but not necessarily to thrive. Our souls are capable, sometimes more capable, of evolving with modest financial resources than lavish ones, even though our culture is based on financial power. This chapter will help guide you to a relationship with money that can foster your soul health instead of weakening it.

ASSESSING YOUR RELATIONSHIP WITH MONEY

Money is not required to buy one necessity of the soul. ~~ Henry David Thoreau

Why are we so easily threatened by money? What makes us feel vulnerable when we think and talk about our finances? What buttons does it push if we think we don't have enough? Is that really a matter of lacking what we need, or is it a matter of trying to keep up with others?

In my mind, few people in our society have a healthy relationship with money. Instead, we fear it—sometimes both having it and not having it. We all dream about having vast financial resources, but what would you do with great wealth if you had it? Would your problems really go away? How many wealthy people do you know of who truly lead a soulful life? Ironically, it is often those with the most money whose lives are the least focused on soul. In fact, they tend to live further and further away from their souls and often get themselves into trouble with the things they bury themselves in—

debt, drugs, empty relationships, extravagant homes, planes, boats, cars and other "toys".

Researchers Paul Piff and Dacher Keltner have offered numerous studies showing that as riches grow, empathy, compassion, and patience for others seems to decline. They found that wealthy people a) tend to perceive that their personal needs are more urgent than others, b) that they experience less compassion for those who are suffering, c) that they are worse at recognizing the emotions of others, and d) that they are less likely to pay attention to those that they are interacting with. Piff and Keltner also showed that having limited financial resources does not lead to selfishness as some might think. In fact, the opposite is true—the upper class is more likely to agree with statements that greed is justifiable, beneficial, and morally defensible. These attitudes toward money were also found to predict the likelihood of engaging in unethical behavior.

EXERCISE

Clearly, our relationship with money has many implications on our experience of the human condition, and thus on our soul. Take a few minutes to consider your relationship with money. Write down your ideas about money as well as a description of how money currently defines you.

Do you have a healthy relationship with money? It may seem odd to refer to your connection with money as a relationship, but in fact, we hold money near and dear—sometimes even more than loved ones. Just as in our human relationships, we may relate to money with issues of trust, guilt, respect (or lack of respect), poor boundaries, and so on. It is almost as if coins and bills hold more power over us than anything else. The energy surrounding money can cause conflict within ourselves and with others, and on a larger scale can cause wars, riots, and other forms of dissension. Even when we feel we have enough money, it can seem to create an invisible protective shield around us—a comfort zone in which we feel protected against illness or other troubles money can't solve.

Like most things, our ideas about money tend to be formed in our early years and often relate to the way we saw our parents deal, or not deal, with money. Until we are financially responsible for ourselves, our relationship with money is usually dictated by those who raised us and how they spent or saved money. In some cases, we grow up witnessing caregivers' unhealthy relationships with money and must change our own ways in order to avoid the same patterns. But until we learn what our souls need in order to truly thrive, our financial health tends to remain shaky.

Following is the Financial Branch of Health Questionnaire. Take a few minutes to complete the survey and explore the aspects of creating a healthier relationship with money for your soul health.

QUESTIONNAIRE FOR THE FINANCIAL BRANCH OF HEALTH

On a scale of 1 to 10, rate the level of your health within each area described. A 10 describes optimal, radiant health, while a 1 describes an almost complete lack of health within the given aspect of the financial branch. Remember, this questionnaire is designed to create a roadmap to overall radiant health. It is not meant to overwhelm you.

Financial Security
1. _____ I feel financially secure.
2. _____ I have enough money to pay my monthly bills.
3. _____ I feel I will always have what I need.
4. _____ I am not stressed about money.
5. _____ Paying bills does not cause me stress.
6. _____ I have enough resources to manage sudden expenses.

Management of Resources
1. _____ I manage money well.
2. _____ I do not live paycheck to paycheck.
3. _____ I am free of debt.
4. _____ I am comfortable with the amount of debt that I have.
5. _____ I pay cash for most purchases.
6. _____ I pay off credit cards each month.
7. _____ I generally know what my monthly expenses will be.
8. _____ I can anticipate when certain extra expenses are approaching.

Spending Habits
1. _____ I buy only items I can afford.
2. _____ Generally, I do not spend beyond my means.
3. _____ I avoid buying things impulsively.
4. _____ I plan for what I purchase.
5. _____ Generally, I follow a weekly or monthly budget.
6. _____ I buy only what I need.

Financial Planning
1. _____ I regularly save for the future.
2. _____ I have planned for retirement from an early age.
3. _____ I have a realistic idea of how much money I will need for retirement.
4. _____ I have a plan for paying off debts.
5. _____ I have a plan for spending and saving.
6. _____ I understand most investment language and terms.
7. _____ I have both short- and long-term financial goals.
8. _____ I know how to save money through tax deductions, tax credits, and so on.

Beliefs About Money
1. _____ My beliefs about money are realistic.
2. _____ I know my financial resources are my responsibility.
3. _____ Others would agree that I am responsible with how I spend money.
4. _____ My idea of success is motivated by more than money.
5. _____ I do not take money for granted.
6. _____ I know that my perception of financial security affects all other aspects of my life.

Unless you are in a career that deals directly with managing financial resources, whether for individuals, banks, corporations, charities, or other groups, it is unlikely that you have thought hard about your own relationship with money, as laid out in the questionnaire above. Even if you work in a career related to accounting or finances, you may not follow your own advice. Many people are surprised by their reactions to the questionnaire. However, when you carefully assess your relationship with money, you will see its impact on the relationship you have with your soul as well.

FINANCIAL SECURITY

My soul whispered that what I really yearned for was not financial security but financial serenity. ~~ Sarah Ban Breathnach

Our perceptions about lack or abundance are at the heart of our need for financial security. But our ideas about what is really necessary can conflict with the needs of our soul. At a basic level, of course, we do need enough resources for our survival, but beyond that we are often fooled by society to think we need more objects, success, or status in order for our souls to thrive. Though certain pleasures and possessions can serve our soul's health, few are necessary for its evolution.

Author Sarah Ban Breathnach, in describing her own struggles with finding financial security, said that the more she focused on "lack" the more depressed she got, and the more depressed she got, the more she continued to focus on what she did not have. This is when she discovered that finding peace within was the key to a healthy relationship with the simple abundance in her life. She recognized that the simplicity in her life was more valuable than vast wealth. She learned to appreciate the simple things in life that brought her joy and went on to become a best-selling author as a result, which brought her more wealth.

Our financial security depends primarily on what we *perceive* our needs to be and whether we believe we have enough money to support them. Many have the resources to meet their needs, but their built-in fears prevent them from attaining them. Others may not have the financial resources to acquire what they think they need, when, in truth, their desired objects are not necessary for their soul's growth and evolution.

What we regard as our genuine needs within our experience of the human condition can be complex, though the needs of the soul are strikingly simple. As humans, we often believe we need many things around us—cars, houses, televisions, cell phones, and so on—to make us feel secure and complete. However, our souls need much less in order to evolve. In fact, we often grow more when faced with the idea of having less. Our feelings and ideas about money, when we examine them closely, can lead us to peace no matter how much or how little we have.

> » What has created your sense of financial security or lack of one?

> » What helps you to feel more peaceful when you think of your resources?

> » What does your soul really need to feel more secure?

MANAGEMENT OF RESOURCES

*It is great wealth to a soul to live frugally with
a contented mind.* ~~ Lucretius

Businesses that help you manage your finances constitute a

multimillion dollar enterprise themselves. So many people have difficulty managing their money that they are willing to pay significant amounts of it to attend programs, buy CDs, videos, and books, and hire financial counselors, coaches, and planners to get a better handle on their resources. What they learn as a result is logical but often does not teach that our relationship with money is what created our problems with management to begin with.

Once again, our upbringing has an effect on how we manage our finances—how we save or spend, how we pay—or don't pay—our bills, and how we acquire and manage debt. If our parents bought more than they could afford, it often means we will do the same. If we grew up with the feeling that there was never enough money, we will also carry that into the future. Unless we examine and are able to change our behavior, we will manage our financial resources like those who raised us.

Managing both our income and our financial output is rather like monitoring our soul health. Like the soul, we need more resources coming in than going out in order to feel comfortable and healthy. When we buy something that is beyond our means, it usually creates an inner discomfort or anxiety. This, of course, is the soul's voice trying to get our attention. Our *dis*-ease which follows an extensive purchase is our inner wisdom cautioning us, often through our buyer's regret. When we listen to it—ideally before we finalize and unwise expense—we are able to make financial choices that align with our soul. In those cases, we feel no discomfort, only contentment.

> » Does your financial management style allow you to feel at ease or cause you discomfort?

> » Do you have a gut feeling that you are not managing your money well? What can you change to align your income and expenditures with the needs of your soul?

» How did you learn to manage your money? Is your method conducive to your soul health?

SPENDING HABITS

Poverty of goods is easily cured; poverty of soul, impossible. ~~ Michel de Montaigne

If we believe we *require* something other than a basic need to survive and thrive, this could indicate an unhealthy soul, especially if what we think we need creates a financial hardship and stress. True, sometimes we have to spend money to heal our souls (for example on physical, emotional, or spiritual therapy, inspiring vacations, restorative retreats, or thought-provoking books) , but this usually doesn't include the extravagances like the most expensive sports cars, high definition televisions, or jewelry.

Our souls are simple; they need very little to thrive. In most cases, it is our dissatisfaction with life that tells us what we "should" have in order to feel better about ourselves and our circumstances. Clearly, though, compulsive shopping or mismanagement of money only erodes our soul health and creates discord in our lives. It creates a battle between our experience of the human condition and our soul.

» Do you often buy more than what you truly need?

» Do you buy things to soothe uncomfortable emotions?

» If you were to look around and ask what you could do without, what would your soul say?

» What do you honestly need around you in order to feel inner peace?

Most of us have more possessions than we will ever really need. But knowing this, and acting accordingly, makes genuine peace—or soul health— possible.

PLANNING FOR THE FUTURE

If you fail to plan, you plan to fail. ~~ Harvey MacKay

Planning of any sort requires an expanded consciousness about the big picture at hand. When it comes to money, our ability to survive and thrive has everything to do with our ability to look ahead, consider our needs and resources, and plan accordingly. Becoming and remaining conscious about our financial health is a key ingredient to an overall sense of well-being which directly affects soul health.

However, the immediacy of our human emotions is a major influence on whether we plan for our financial future. Our desire for instant gratification often dictates whether we tuck that extra five dollars aside or spend it on coffee, whether we buy that new television for the big game, or save the extra hundreds of dollars for a rainy day.

Saving for the future does much more for us than protect us from financial crises we can't foresee. It also protects our soul. When we plan for possible hard times by saving money and investing for retirement, this is nothing less than an insurance policy for our daily lives as well as our souls. Deep down, we know we will weather life's storms better if we know that we have a financial cushion against hard times or emergencies. In this way, not only is our human condition cared for, but also our soul. As we work on this in tandem with our soul's desires and needs, we can rest easy about practical matters and also with a deep inner peace. We can continue to evolve regardless of financial challenges because we are prepared for them.

This forethought solidifies the foundation that not only will we take care of our basic needs, but also foster our soul's need to grow.

» What is your philosophy on saving money?

» How do you feel about saving for the future?

» Are you susceptible to impulse buying or do you plan for your future first?

» Is your soul at ease with how you plan for the future?

BELIEFS ABOUT MONEY

Ordinary riches can be stolen; real riches cannot.
In your soul are infinitely precious things that
cannot be taken from you. ~~ Oscar Wilde

It may seem odd to consider our beliefs about money, but we all hold them whether they are healthy or not. Whether we believe that money is good or evil has much to do with this. Our beliefs about money are influenced by our childhood experiences of watching our elders grapple with money issues; they are further affected by other ways we have learned to grapple with them for ourselves. Though money indeed doesn't grow on trees, many people act as if it does.

Ideas of success, financial responsibility, an appreciation of your resources, a realistic viewpoint about money, and your conscious understanding of the overall impact of your financial choices on the rest of your life—all of these are woven into your overall feelings and ideas about money. If you remain mindful of these issues and consciously develop and change them as necessary, you are more likely to have a healthy financial branch of soul health.

In other words, financial responsibility relates directly to responsibility for your soul. A later chapter will explore the idea of soul stewardship as your personal responsibility toward caring for your soul's health. Similarly, financial stewardship, in the form of a plan to manage your resources responsibly, helps to build a foundation for your soul's health and evolution. Financial insecurity, like any other stress related to the human condition, inhibits the soul's growth.

» How do you define financial success?

» How did you learn (or not learn) to appreciate your financial resources?

» Are you a good steward of your resources?

SACRED FINANCE

Man cannot be satisfied by wealth. ~~ Katha Upanishad

There is nothing sacred about money itself—sacredness lies in the meaning we ascribe to it. Often it is in having less, not more, that we build the platform on which our souls can grow.

In his book *Sacred Economics*, Charles Eisenstein outlines the history of money as well as the influence money has had on our overall sense of separation from ourselves, each other, and the world at large. Eisenstein writes about how communities of the world have become fractured by getting lost in concepts of money, and points out how money, rather than an inner life, has become the focal point for most people. He emphasizes that both the meaning and power of money have morphed into ends in their own right rather than the means of supplementing growth and consciousness.

Another author, Lynne Twist, provides a philosophical view of money through the eyes of both the rich and the poor. Her book, *The*

Soul of Money offers a broad view concerning ideas about scarcity, prosperity, abundance, and success. She interviews everyone from Mother Teresa, who dedicated her life to aiding the poor, and to others who are vastly wealthy. In her work as a global fundraiser, she has woven her experiences into her writing and captured the essence of everyone's longing for financial security.

Both books offer views that can be helpful in developing your own financial well-being and applying it to soul health.

SUCCESS OR SIGNIFICANCE?

People do not care how much you know until they know how much you care. ~~ John Maxwell

International speaker and leadership expert, John Maxwell, addresses the fundamental differences between success and significance, noting that true significance has nothing to do with money, whereas success is often defined by it. Instead, significance has much more to do with our ability to make meaning in our lives through constructive efforts to improve the world around us. Because many who become extremely wealthy also tend to become more and more focused on money, as an end itself, Maxwell strongly advises staying focused on your impact on others as you attain your financial goals.

The idea of success as opposed to significance is important to the health of the soul. Although we need money to survive, our soul is fed best by the meaning we create in our lives and the lives of others. The soul is all about finding meaning in the world. And when we remain focused on altruism we fuel our soul and are able to spread ever widening benefit to others.

The soul knows when it is doing its job for the world. It knows when it is following its calling or purpose. Little of this has to do with money; much more of it involves the deep satisfaction we, and therefore our soul, receive from making even a small positive difference in the world.

One doesn't have to become another Mother Teresa in order to experience soul health. What is important is a commitment to a balanced and healthy understanding of money and your own financial health. A better relationship with money will not only serve your soul, but also lead to good acts for others.

» What can you do to develop a better relationship with money?

» How does your financial health impact your soul?

» Are you more concerned with success or with significance?

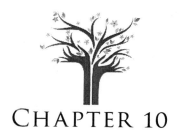

CHAPTER 10

SPIRITUAL HEALTH:
SOUL-BASED LIVING

To be rooted is perhaps the most important and least recognized need of the human soul. ~~ Simone Weil

Philosopher Simone Weil reflected on the importance of feeling "rooted" in life in order to fulfill the deepest needs of the soul. This rootedness comes from *knowing* your soul and aligning with its most essential needs and values. As mentioned in previous chapters, to know your soul is to know true health. Truly knowing your soul requires an exploration of the deepest values and meanings by which we live. This internal inventory, or journey, allows us to discover our inner essence and helps us to align our daily lives with our innermost ally to create soul health.

What anchors, grounds, or roots you? What ideas, thoughts, people, places, and activities help you to feel at peace in your life? What feelings, thoughts, or sensations let you know when you aren't at ease or balanced? What inspires you—and what does not? Do you see the world as part of your path or journey? How aware are you of your soul and the wisdom it has to offer?

Spiritual health is integral to our overall health and well-being whether or not we acknowledge this. We all seek inner peace and recognize when something in our lives is blocking it. This disequilibrium is our warning sign that our life is somehow misaligned with our soul, in which case other parts of our life—other branches—become disturbed or unbalanced. Paying attention to this internal alert system helps us proactively balance our lives, and more effectively and consistently experience soul health. However, ignoring this integral aspect of our health will only inhibit our sense of peace, our healing, and our soul's evolution.

This chapter shows how spiritual health is essential to creating radiant health. It emphasizes the difference between spirituality and religion and discusses how even our healthcare systems are beginning to see that it is important to integrate spiritual health into overall care. This chapter also explores various dimensions of spiritual health and stresses that spirituality is a very personal process, one that is unique to each individual. It not only paves the way for radiant health but anchors it so strongly that nothing can truly disturb it, once its foundation is defined.

LIVING THROUGH THE SOUL

Soul-based living requires an awareness and conscious appreciation of how our inner wisdom guides our lives. This lets us put wisdom to good use in our day-to-day experiences, something we could not do without the little voice within us that tells us whether or not something feels right in our lives. For example, when we feel unsettled or stressed, our soul—or inner wisdom— tells us to seek peace through whatever means will fulfill this need (time alone, exercise, reading, spending time in nature). This voice lets us know when we are not at peace and/or when we have strayed from the path that leads to peace in our lives. If we pay attention to this message, we can become more grounded or rooted, however tumultuous the circumstances of our human condition may be.

Spirituality relates to "that which affects or relates to the human spirit" and sets people on an inner path that leads them to discover the essence of their being. In relation to consciousness, our spiritual path is the journey we accept as we discover how the struggles in our human condition fit into a grander scheme. In other words, spirituality is an experience of an expanded reality—our highest consciousness— that allows us to identify our place in the world and arrive at peace concerning our life's purpose, our mission, and our path in general. The spiritual branch of the Soul Health Model emphasizes our active role in creating this awareness and path.

Spirituality is often described as holding a belief in a power greater than ourselves, and we achieve spiritual health when this belief leads to inner peace, a sense of our purpose as humans, and an awareness of our spirit separate from our human qualities. There are many ways to seek this internally heightened life, including prayer, meditation, ritual, and other forms of grounding in spirit that will be discussed later.

Modern definitions of spirituality derive from the words "inspire" or "in spirit" and those who are seen as highly spiritual are often viewed as inspirational or enlightened. So it only makes sense that our innermost voice, if we listen for it, can serve as our ultimate inspiration for our soul health. When any of the other branches of health wither, it is often because we lack inspiration in general. This is a sign that we have lost touch with our soul and more absorbed by the human condition than in our spirit condition—our soul.

When we are not inspired by life, how do we feel? Bored? Uninterested? Bummed out? In any case, we can bet that our health is anything but radiant. It is when we live through our soul that we feel fully engaged in our everyday lives.

What inspires you? What keeps you from feeling bored with life? What kinds of thoughts, feelings, or experiences nourish you at a deeper level than any food ever could? Is there something that never fails to bring you peace? When was the last time you took the time to explore your deepest values and how you derive meaning from life?

Living through your soul brings an unmistakable awareness of how life works and how it pieces together, offering meaning at every moment and through every experience. In this way, consciousness is all about spirituality and spirituality is all about consciousness. One cannot be spiritually healthy without being conscious of one's place and one's impact on the world. To be spiritually healthy is to recognize that we are all on the same journey, no matter what gender, religion, race, or difference we may have with others. Being conscious of this *is* a spiritual experience.

With regard to spiritual health, once a person experiences a true sense of spirituality they become forever able to recognize when they no longer feel this way— they recognize when they aren't living through the soul. They feel unwell or empty regardless of their physical health. Something vital seems to be missing. Our job is to find our sense of spirit, because that balances the rest of our soul health and creates a more radiant way of living.

Although the Soul Health Model itself has spiritual implications, it is the intentional commitment to a spiritually healthy life that allows the rest of the branches of health to thrive and sets the stage for our souls to evolve. As humans, we must work in tandem with our soul to create a healthy existence, and we cannot accomplish this without a personal dedication to focusing on, and satisfying our unique spiritual needs.

Following is the Spiritual Branch of Health Questionnaire. As you rate your responses, consider what you can do to enhance your spiritual wellbeing with respect to the other branches of health.

QUESTIONNAIRE FOR THE SPIRITUAL BRANCH OF HEALTH

On a scale of 1 to 10, rate the level of your health within each area described. A 10 describes optimal, radiant health, while a 1 describes an almost complete lack of health within the given aspect of the spiritual branch. Remember, this questionnaire is designed to create a roadmap to overall radiant health. It is not meant to overwhelm you.

Sense of Inner Peace
1. _____ Spirituality is important to me.
2. _____ I have good spiritual wellness.
3. _____ I have inner peace.
4. _____ I actively seek ways to create inner peace.
5. _____ I can find inner peace without using unhealthy substances.
6. _____ I know when I need to re-center or ground myself.
7. _____ Feeling inner peace allows me to live my life more effectively.
8. _____ I know what it takes to help me find inner peace.

Beliefs about Spirituality and Religion
1. _____ I know the difference between spirituality and religion.
2. _____ I feel good about my spiritual and/or religious beliefs.
3. _____ I feel safe sharing my beliefs with others.
4. _____ I find peace in my spiritual beliefs.
5. _____ I am clear about my spiritual beliefs.
6. _____ My spiritual beliefs are healthy for me and others around me.
7. _____ I find meaning and purpose through my spiritual beliefs.
8. _____ My spiritual beliefs do not leave me feeling conflicted or guilty.

Spiritual Practices
1. _____ I actively practice my spiritual beliefs.
2. _____ I practice my beliefs on a daily basis.
3. _____ The people in my life support my spiritual practices.
4. _____ My spiritual practices enhance inner peace and strength.
5. _____ I know when I need to spend more time in my spiritual practices to feel more balanced or well.
6. _____ I actively seek to learn more about my spirituality.
7. _____ My spiritual activities are an important part of my daily life.

World View
1. _____ I accept others' spiritual beliefs.
2. _____ I recognize that it is okay to have different spiritual beliefs from others.
3. _____ I am open to learning about other people's spiritual beliefs and practices.
4. _____ I do not impose my spiritual beliefs on others.
5. _____ I believe I am part of a larger whole or picture.
6. _____ I know I can learn from others' spiritual beliefs and practices, even if they aren't my own.

Soul Awareness
1. _____ I know clarity increases when I listen to my soul.
2. _____ I accept troublesome events as opportunities for soul growth.
3. _____ I am aware of what my soul needs in order to feel spiritually well.
4. _____ When I listen, I can hear my inner voice in every moment.
5. _____ I know when my soul feels stagnant and when it is evolving.

What did you learn from this questionnaire about your spiritual health? What areas do you need to explore further? Which parts of your life give you a sense of peace and which ones interfere with that?

Much like the other branches of health, the spiritual branch is multidimensional—possibly even more than the others. Certainly this branch affects all others, but not everyone may understand what it means to be spiritual or spiritually-minded. Many people believe that a formal religious belief system is necessary to spirituality. This is true for some, but for many, spirituality arises simply from understanding what creates inner peace and meaning in their lives. For them, this is what it means to live in spirit—to live through their soul. Awareness of the spiritual branch, that is, a conscious effort to see soul health as an interconnected whole, allows us a deeper fulfillment.

INNER PEACE

Nowhere can man find a quieter or more untroubled retreat than in his own soul. ~~ Marcus Aurelius

Inner peace is described as a state of being mentally and spiritually centered and calm even in the face of discord or stress. This might seem impossible given that the circumstances of our human condition present many opportunities to become enveloped by the stressors of everyday life. Finding this inner equilibrium, regardless of the turmoil we may experience, is considered to be the ultimate consciousness. When a person can reach this level of enlightenment, they are clearly on a steady path to their soul's evolution. Many spiritual traditions, including Buddhism and Hinduism, emphasize the attainment of inner peace as the key element of daily practice. Much like spirituality itself, finding inner peace is an individual process— that which brings peace is often unique to the individual. However, common to all is the desire to reach this internal solace.

> » When was the last time you felt complete inner peace?

> » What circumstances allowed you to reach this state of being?

> » What happened to interrupt your peace?

> » Is there one thing you could do every day to instill a more permanent sense of inner peace in your life?

BELIEFS ABOUT SPIRITUALITY AND RELIGION

All are parts of one stupendous whole. Whose body
Nature is, and God the soul. ~~ Alexander Pope

Religion and spirituality are not synonymous; in fact, they differ in both meaning and practice. The word spirituality stems from the word inspire, while the original meaning of the word religion is somewhat obscure. Currently, the word religion refers to a set of concepts that are held in common and practiced by a community, much like moral law. Although many think the terms are highly related, it is not necessary to be religious in order to be spiritual, nor vice versa. In fact, the two are altogether separate.

Religion tends to be somewhat exclusive—separating us from other formal belief systems—, while spirituality is inclusive in nature—acknowledging that although each person is on their own path, we are all on a similar journey of self-discovery. Religion is seen as a way of *doing*—following a specific dogma or set of rituals—, while spirituality is most often described as a way of *being*—experiencing life and its meaning through every breath, thought, and action.

Therefore, to be religious is not necessarily to be spiritual, and to be spiritual is not necessarily to be religious. You can have both together, or you can have one without the other.

The core of spiritual health is that you feel at ease and comfortable with your belief system, whether religious, spiritual, or both. If you have thoughts or behaviors that conflict with your beliefs, you are likely to feel some anxiety and discomfort. People often feel a sense of disharmony as they grow away from the teaching of their families of origin or their cultures in which they were raised. Such a split is sometimes necessary on the path to your soul's evolution. The primary goal of spiritual health is to feel at peace with your beliefs and allow yourself the open and free expression of them. This is not always easy, but the process is important as we evolve toward our strongest inner truth and advance toward our soul health.

» How comfortable are you with your belief system?

» Can you openly express your beliefs?

» Do you hold any negative emotions related to your spiritual beliefs?

» What can you do to gain a clearer understanding of your spirituality?

SPIRITUAL PRACTICES

When you do things from your soul you feel a river moving in you, a joy. When action comes from another section, the feeling disappears. ~~ Rumi

Nothing is more personal than our spiritual practices. While religious activities tend to be performed in groups and led by a priest or minister, our spirituality is often practiced alone. Because spirituality is more a way of *being* than *doing*, our moments of inspiration can come at any time, and our questions, prayers, and pleas to a higher power are at least as likely to be offered alone as in a group of like-minded others.

When we are committed to a spiritual practice, we tend to feel more engaged in life; we find more meaning, live with greater gratitude, and remain more conscious of how we affect the world and how it affects us. Though spiritual practices vary widely (prayer, meditation, yoga, tai chi, ritual, singing, chanting, dancing, communing with nature, reading, discussion), it is our active participation in them that supports our spiritual health and centers us in that place of inner peace. Just like engaging in physical activity for fitness, our engagement in spiritual practice strengthens and enhances our spiritual branch of health, which in turn, enhances our overall soul health.

» How often do you engage in individual spiritual practices?

» When do your most inspirational moments occur?

» How do you actively find spiritual meaning?

» What activities do you incorporate in your spiritual practices to feel more grounded?

WORLDVIEW

Say not, "I have found the truth," but rather, "I have found a truth." Say not, "I have found the path of the soul." Say rather, "I have met the soul walking upon my path." For the soul walks upon all paths. ~~ Kahlil Gibran, *The Prophet.*

Having a healthy spiritual worldview means not only that you value your beliefs, but also that you accept and even welcome others' as well. Though the Ten Commandments tell us to love thy neighbor, endless wars and disagreements have erupted over differing religious beliefs.

Religious or spiritual prejudices, like many others, signal that we are not completely at ease with our own beliefs. Highly spiritual people have no need to judge others; instead, they welcome differing ideas and cherish the opportunity to commune with others regardless. Enlightened individuals also have no need to impose their spiritual ideas on others, for they see each person's beliefs as part of the greater whole or good. In fact, highly spiritual people tend to be more curious and willing to learn about others' belief systems and are generally more open and eager to integrating new ideas into their own beliefs.

> » What biases do you hold about other belief systems than your own?

> » How do you judge others based on their beliefs?

> » When was the last time you willingly learned something about another's belief system?

> » In what ways would expanding your own worldview create more inner peace?

SOUL AWARENESS

*Put your ear down close to your soul and
listen hard.* ~~ Anne Sexton

Most of us are not taught to listen to our soul, though it is our most precious ally. Awareness of our soul often comes naturally when we are very young, yet this connection fades due to enculturation. We begin to think and act like others instead of interpreting and living from our inner voice. How different would life be if we were taught from our earliest years to listen to that voice?

Soul awareness requires us to acknowledge that we have an inner voice, that it has much wisdom to share, and that we have deep, spiritual needs that must be fulfilled in order to experience radiant health and inner peace. This awareness is what leads us down the path of evolution, where we welcome each and every situation as an opportunity to learn and grow. This consciousness also allows us to apply meaning and purpose to matters related to our human condition, which elevates us to living in spirit—or through our soul— as well. This attentiveness to our soul also lets us recognize when we feel off base or unclear; it stimulates our need to go within to find the clarity we need in order to grow. Soul awareness, an aspect of health, is the key measure of radical consciousness; it is the most necessary ingredient of soul health—simply to be aware, and then to act on our awareness to honor our soul.

> »   When did you first become aware of your soul?

> »   When did you first lose awareness of your soul, once you had it?

> »   What needs to happen for you to develop a stronger awareness of your inner ally?

> »   How does your soul awareness inform you that you need to do something differently to achieve soul health? (Change a belief, behavior, or pattern?)

> »   When do you hear your soul most clearly?

PERSONALIZING YOUR PEACE

*All things must come to the soul from its roots, from
where it is planted.* ~~ Saint Teresa of Avila

Religion requires believers to follow a specific set of beliefs and practices, both in their private lives and within a group setting. Spirituality, though, is completely unique *to* the individual—created *by* the individual! Because each soul is like no other, we must feed or calm our own according to its particular needs. Some people find a sense of peace in nature, while others develop soul consciousness through music, art, silence, or solitude.

No two souls are alike. This makes it impossible for two identical forms of spirituality to exist. The beauty of this is that each of us has the option and ability to completely design our own path to inner peace. Each road looks and feels different. We may share similar beliefs and engage in similar spiritual practices with others, but because each soul reflects the unique person holding it, only that person will know what truly brings them inner solace and soul health.

This is where many people feel challenged by a set of beliefs meant to serve everyone, as in organized religions. They may practice their particular religion but still hold their own beliefs about some or all of the concepts. An internal struggle can ensue when a person reaches a level of soul awareness that conflicts with the beliefs of the group at large. Believe it or not, there is actually a psychological diagnosis (simply called "Religious and Spiritual Problems") for this inner turmoil since many people experience disturbing guilt or fear for questioning their beliefs. The addition of this diagnosis marked a significant breakthrough by acknowledging that spiritual emergencies and crises may occur in the process of growth and change. Given that some religions strongly discourage individual thought about core concepts, departing from the accepted doctrine can greatly challenge a person's ideas about the human condition and therefore distress their soul.

Finding your personal peace means coming to terms with what fits your soul, then setting out to create the belief system that allows your soul to grow. Incidentally, this personalized path more often complements than denies the person's formal religion, in effect, blending group practice with an adapted private spiritual practice. Inevitably, this blend serves to heighten an individual's soul health because it is then tailored to the person's specific truth. This kind of customization serves to promote the soul's evolution.

SPIRITUAL HEALTH AND HEALING

*With all your science—can you tell how it is, and whence it is,
that light comes into the soul?* ~~ Henry David Thoreau

Science has long disassociated itself from spirituality and religion. However, it seems to be coming full circle as hundreds of research articles now note the importance of spiritual health in the lives and recoveries of medical patients.

Eighty-one percent of individuals report that their spirituality is their primary coping mechanism when they are sick. Further research indicates that 94 percent of spiritually-inclined patients wish that spirituality would be addressed during their doctor visits, while less than ten percent of physicians actually do so. Despite this lack of formal attention in medical care, research shows that spirituality has a positive influence overall on health because it improves coping, increases social support, promotes healthy behaviors, reduces anxiety and depression, creates a positive attitude toward healing, increases survival rates, speeds up recovery, reduces regret, and provides greater overall satisfaction with life. In contrast, those who do not have a spiritual life tend to have more negative health outcomes.

Other research shows that faith increases the body's resistance to stress, a feeling of hope tends to boost immunity and extend life span, and forgiveness decreases stress hormones, thus enhancing overall beneficial health outcomes. The research also shows that people who pray regularly feel greater peace and have healthier outcomes overall. It is becoming harder and harder for healthcare professionals to deny the importance of integrating spiritual health into their treatment of patients. If spirituality was more fully incorporated, both healthcare and the response to it would change dramatically.

Whether medical practice directly integrates spirituality or not, it is clear that most people who hold strong spiritual beliefs rely on it while coping with illness, often with great effectiveness. In fact, the earliest medical professionals were priests, shamans, medicine men/women, and natural healers, not scientifically trained practitioners. Even today, in many native cultures and holistic health environments, help for physical ailments still entails a visit to a spiritually-trained or "chosen" healer.

Regardless of your belief system, spiritual health is clearly integral to healing from illness and is an essential aspect in its prevention. Your willingness to pay attention to sickness, understand the message from your soul, and exercise your spirituality to cope and heal is a measure of your spiritual health and allows your consciousness to deepen along with your soul health. It is impossible to deny the enhanced vitality that arises when inner peace develops through the evolution of the soul.

> » How does spirituality influence your healing?

> » How does it help to create meaning in your experience of illness?

> » What other branches of health are influenced by your spiritual branch, and vice versa?

CHAPTER 11

SEXUAL HEALTH:
FROM INTIMACY TO ECSTASY

Sex is God's joke on human beings. ~~ Bette Davis

There is nothing like sex to complicate relationships. These intimate acts can draw two people together or push them apart. Each person's experience of sexual intimacy is as unique as that person's soul. Everyone ascribes a different, multi-layered meaning to sex based on their beliefs, upbringing, attitudes, and experiences—none of which may be soulful at all. All of these influence a person's experience of intimacy and ultimately their soul health.

Most health and wellness models discuss sex only briefly as one small element of overall physical health. However, in my work as a psychologist, it is clear that sexual health deserves much more than a cursory glance. Our knowledge, experiences, and the meanings we apply to sex are all critical in the quest for radiant health.

This chapter explores many facets of the sexual branch of health, including what constitutes a healthy sexual relationship, how our sex life—or lack of one—affects other aspects of soul health, and how unresolved sexual trauma can inhibit our overall health and our soul's evolution altogether.

Soulful Sex

Spiritual relationship is far more precious than physical. Physical relationship divorced from spiritual is body without soul. ~~ Mohandas Gandhi

Sex is a powerful force in human life. It not only expands the population, it also greatly affects and even alters our experience of the human condition. Whether you have too much, too little, or just enough sex, you can be sure that this branch of soul health affects all others. A study by David Blanchflower of Dartmouth College and Andrew Oswald of the University of Warwick indicates that the happiest people, in general, are those who engage in sex most often. The study reported that sex is such a strong and positive factor in the happiness equation that the researchers estimated that, for many people, increasing intercourse from once a month to once a week would generate an increase in happiness equivalent to receiving a $50,000 raise in annual income. While the importance of sex differs from one person to another, the study does imply that healthy sexual activity can enhance overall well-being.

On the other hand, it is widely known that everyday stress, anxiety, and depression can also result in sexual dysfunction or disinterest. This is partly because these conditions decrease sexual hormones, lower serotonin levels, deplete energy, and intensify worrisome thoughts and negative thinking. Unfortunately, many antidepressants—which, of course, are meant to offset these emotional concerns—tend to change brain chemistry in such a way as to diminish blood flow to the sex organs, thus interfering with sexual health even more. Even if a person feels aroused, he or she may not be able to perform. This, of course, can lead to even greater sexual dysfunction and result in feelings of inadequacy or inhibition.

Many other factors influence the health of a person's sex life. Society itself has great impact on people's sexual attitudes and experiences. Impulsive, irresponsible and empty sexual encounters are everywhere in the media (television, movies, magazines, advertisements, internet content). This exposure contributes to the alarming increase in sexual addictions, which now affects one in seven people. Also, statistically speaking, reports of sexual traumas have become nearly epidemic. One-third of girls and women and one-fifth of boys and men suffer sexual abuse, and one-fourth of women are raped during their lives. The impact on sexual health is widespread throughout the branches of soul health.

Many other aspects of the human condition can greatly affect sexual health. Grief, economic concerns, additions to the family, moving to a new home, job stress or change, spiritual or religious concerns, communication issues, physical or emotional issues, and lack of time for leisure or fun can all cause problems in the sexual branch of health. As a result of other life factors, one in five women and one in ten men report that sex gives them no pleasure. Our ability to experience a healthy sex life is complex and awareness of what influences our sexual health is important in balancing our overall well-being.

Making love makes us more vulnerable than any other interaction we will ever have with another human being—it can also be the most soulful encounter shared with another person. Many factors play a part in whether your sexual branch is healthy. Wendy Maltz, a certified sex therapist, clinical social worker, and author, outlines five key aspects of healthy sexuality: consent, equality, respect, trust and safety.

Consent means you are free and comfortable in choosing whether or not to engage in sexual activity with a partner. Consent also implies that you and your partner make a conscious and informed decision to engage in sexual activity and that either one of you can change your mind and stop the sexual activity at any time.

Equality allows both people to feel personal power, with neither one dominating or intimidating the other before, during, or after sexual activity.

Respect is present when you and your partner have positive regard for yourselves and each other, not only through sexual intimacy but in how you treat each other at all times.

Trust is based on both people accepting and showing sensitivity to each other's needs and vulnerabilities.

Safety means that you and your partner feel no emotional or physical risk or danger as you engage in sex and that you are comfortable and assertive about where, when, and how the sexual activity takes place. You also have no fear of negative consequences such as unwanted pregnancy or sexually transmitted disease.

When you think about these five characteristics of healthy sexual relationships, you can't help but imagine a soulful bond with a partner. Sadly, though, how often are all these necessary conditions portrayed in our culture? The depictions of sexual encounters in books, magazines, television, movies, and the internet are too often not examples of soulful interactions. Instead, the image of sex we receive is often one of merchandizing goods, sensationalizing the plot of a movie, or exposing a betrayal or scandal on a talk show. Our ideas of normal sexual changes across our lifespan have also been skewed by the misuse and overuse of drugs for erectile dysfunction and other naturally-occurring sexual concerns that emerge as we age. Somehow these natural changes have become pathologized rather than acknowledged as a normal part of aging.

Following is the Questionnaire for the Sexual Branch of Health. As you answer the questions, consider the soulfulness of your sexual health as well as how this branch affects your overall soul health.

Questionnaire for the Sexual Branch of Health

On a scale of 1 to 10, rate the level of your health within each area described. A 10 describes optimal, radiant health, while a 1 describes an almost complete lack of health within the given aspect of the sexual branch. Remember, this questionnaire is designed to create a roadmap to overall radiant health. It is not meant to overwhelm you.

Knowledge
1. _____ I know what it means to engage in sex.
2. _____ I am knowledgeable about sexual practices.
3. _____ I am knowledgeable about sexual anatomy and sexual responses.
4. _____ I know my body and its sexual responses.
5. _____ I understand how I developed my beliefs and attitudes about sex.
6. _____ I know what I like and don't like when it comes to sex.
7. _____ I know how to prevent an unwanted pregnancy.
8. _____ I know what a sexually-transmitted disease is and how to prevent it.

Safety
1. _____ I know what safe sex is.
2. _____ I engage only in safe sex.
3. _____ I never wonder if I have been unsafe with a sexual partner.
4. _____ I have received adequate education about safe sex.
5. _____ I take precautions to prevent unwanted pregnancies.
6. _____ I take precautions to prevent sexually transmitted diseases.
7. _____ I always talk to sex partners about their sexual health before engaging in sex with them.

Security
1. _____ I feel emotionally secure when engaging in sex.
2. _____ I feel physically secure when engaging in sex.
3. _____ I have sex only with partners I trust.
4. _____ I can communicate freely with my partner(s) about sex.
5. _____ I know and respect my own sexual boundaries.
6. _____ I know and respect the sexual boundaries of others.
7. _____ I feel good about my sexuality.
8. _____ I feel good about expressing myself sexually with my partner(s).

Beliefs about Sex
1. _____ I have healthy beliefs about sex.
2. _____ I do not feel guilty about sex.
3. _____ I do not feel ashamed of sex.
4. _____ My beliefs about sex do not interfere with how I feel about other aspects of my life.
5. _____ I enjoy sex.
6. _____ I feel good about my sex life.

Past Experiences
1. _____ I have consented to all of my sexual experiences.
2. _____ I have only positive memories of my sexual experiences.
3. _____ My past sexual experiences have not negatively affected my sex life.
4. _____ I have sought help to resolve issues related to past negative sexual experiences.
5. _____ I feel at peace with all past sexual experiences.

KNOWLEDGE

Love's mysteries in souls do grow, but yet the
body is his book. ~~ John Donne

"What you don't know won't hurt you" does not apply to sex. However, few people receive an adequate sex education, let alone see good role models for a healthy sexual relationship. What we learn about sex usually comes from our peers, television, movies, books, and magazines and the proverbial birds-and-bees talk from parents is usually greatly abbreviated or absent altogether.

George Bernard Shaw expressed his concerns for our youth's lack of sexual education in stating, "Instruction in sex is as important as instruction in food; yet not only are our adolescents not taught the physiology of sex, but never warned that the strongest sexual attraction may exist between persons so incompatible in tastes and capacities that they could not endure living together for a week much less a lifetime."

Certainly, a general understanding of sex is necessary for a satisfying relationship; however, it takes much more than this to create a bond conducive to soul health. As mentioned in the chapters on the social and interpersonal branches, our relationships often teach us our most vital life lessons. Therefore, knowledge of your needs for sex and intimacy will take you to more conscious unions with others. For this to happen, sexual health must include knowledge not only of the mechanics of sex, but also of the emotional, spiritual, and interpersonal factors that can affect our sexual health.

» Where did you learn about sex? Do you trust that these sources or people provided good and accurate information?

» What questions do you have about sex that were never addressed or answered?

» How have you expanded your knowledge about sex on your own?

SAFETY

For the first time in history, sex is more dangerous than the cigarette afterward. ~~Jay Leno

Given the high rates of sexual assault and sexually transmitted diseases (1 in 4 people in each case), one cannot stress enough the importance of safety. However, safety in a soulful sexual relationship has just as much to do with emotional security as with possible physical risks.

As noted in the chapter on the interpersonal branch of health, several factors are essential for all emotionally healthy relationships; the same applies to emotional safety in sexual relationships. Communication, healthy boundaries, personal integrity, equality, respect, and unconditionality toward your partner's needs and insecurities all play a part in developing a healthy sexual relationship. If any of these are missing from your interpersonal relationship, they will also be lacking in your sexual relationship.

Many people experience close calls in their sexual relationships, fearing they will become pregnant or contract an STD. In the human condition, our physical enjoyment sometimes overrides the need to take precautions, but giving in to the moment can undermine our sense of physical safety. Appropriate precautions, thus, guard your physical, emotional, and ultimately your soul health. Remaining aware of unnecessary risks can safeguard you from potentially traumatic sexual events. According to the National Institutes of Health, more than half of all sexual assaults occur when the perpetrator, the victim, or both are under the influence of alcohol. Awareness about the effects of alcohol on your own behavior may prevent unwanted sexual advances by others.

> » What safety precautions do you need to protect your sexual health?

> » What concerns do you have for safety related to sex in your life?

> » How often do you re-evaluate your safe-sex practices?

SECURITY

Boundaries are to protect life, not to limit pleasures. ~~ Edwin Louis Cole

While physical safety is imperative in creating a healthy sexual relationship, emotional security is also important in enjoying healthy, soulful sex. Even so, far too many people engage in sex even when they don't feel emotionally safe or spiritually connected with their partners. Interactions like these inevitably impact your overall radiant health because they dishonor your deepest ally—your soul. In my psychotherapy practice, I often hear stories from individuals who feel pressured to engage in sex to make their partners happy, regardless of their own sexual interest or emotional safety at the time. To experience full sexual health, one must not dishonor oneself in the process.

Emotional security in a soulful relationship requires open and honest communication with your partner about your needs, likes, dislikes, and interest in sex at any given time. If ever you feel pressured or disrespected, then the partnership is not soul-based, and further mistrust and insecurity are likely. If you cannot honor your own boundaries, you cannot fully experience healthy sex, nor can you create a soulful relationship with yourself or others.

»   How does emotional security affect your sexual health?

»   What do you need from your partner in order to feel emotionally secure when engaging in sex?

»   How openly can you speak to your partner about your needs?

»   How soulful is your relationship with regard to security?

BELIEFS ABOUT SEX

Sex relieves tension—love causes it. ~~ Woody Allen

As it does with most other things, our early upbringing influences our ideas and beliefs about sex. In addition, our sexual beliefs are shaped by everything from culture, religion, societal values, gender roles, and the media as well as beliefs and attitudes passed on by both our elders and our peers. Sexual trauma— abuse, molestation, assault, inappropriate exposure to sexual content— tends to alter our ideas about sexual health. In fact, it is difficult to find anyone these days who doesn't have some sort of sexual glitch or hang-up. In western culture, this is partly because sex continues to be a taboo subject despite its widespread presence in the media.

If shame enters the picture when you are thinking or talking about sex, it is important to take a look at your beliefs and how they were formed. It is not unusual for years and even decades to go by in a relationship with neither person talking about their beliefs regarding sex. People in soulful relationships are able to discuss their thoughts and feelings about sex openly and can explore flawed or unhealthy beliefs in order to improve the health of the union.

- » How were your ideas or beliefs about sex formed?
- » Who did you—or can you—talk to about these beliefs?
- » In your relationship, when was the last time you talked about your sexual beliefs?
- » How have your beliefs changed? How would you like them to change?

PAST EXPERIENCES

The tragedy of sexual intercourse is the perpetual virginity of the soul. ~~ William B. Yeats

All of our past experiences bring us to the present; and unfortunately, some of these may have diminished our ability to fully engage in healthy sexual relationships. Emotional or physical abandonment by parents in our childhood may have led us to forge unhealthy bonds as adults. Inappropriate early sexual encounters may have taught us that love *is* sex, not just one component of love. Rigid beliefs we were taught as children may infuse sex with shame. Sexual trauma may make us feel "dirty" even though the offensive act was completely out of our control.

Whatever our past, there is no way it cannot affect our present and our future; and this goes for sexual health as much as for soul health. Understanding and healing our past—a main concept of the Soul Health Model—will allow us to develop our overall radiant health.

» What sexual traumas or experiences do you need to resolve or heal?

» How do these experiences play a part in your current sexual health?

» How open are you with your partner about these events?

» Have you considered seeking professional assistance in resolving these?

SEX AND SOUL HEALTH

All aspects of soul health directly affect the sexual branch, but there is a reciprocal effect as well. Many studies show positive impacts of sex on general physical health. A healthy sex life has been shown to improve cardiac health, increase immunity, decrease the likelihood of strokes and prostate cancer, reduce generalized pain, and improve sleep. From the psychological perspective, sex has also been shown to decrease stress, improve self-esteem, and improve intimacy between partners.

On the other hand, compromised soul health— or a lack of balance in life— is strongly tied to sex difficulties, especially in today's world. Growing numbers of people find that their sex life suffers due to long hours at work, leaving less energy for sexual intimacy. It is also not uncommon for couples to experience low libido following the birth of a child because their new role as parents is often stressful and exhausting.

Endless other factors contribute to sexual health concerns as well—anxiety, depression, relationship issues, work stress, grief, physical ailments, changes in household status (moves, children entering or leaving the home, income fluctuations, etc.), and the natural changes that come as we move through the life cycle. The challenge, as in all other aspects of health, is to explore which other branches of the human condition are contributing to your experience of sexual health. Whether our lack of sexual health is physically, emotionally, spiritually, intellectually or other-based, reaching an understanding about the connection between sexual health and the rest of the branches will enhance our ability to engage in and enjoy soulful sex. As you explore the Soul Health Model further, you will see how the dots connect and how to rebalance all aspects of health over time.

» What would help make sex more soulful in your life?

» Which other branches of soul health do you need address in order to enhance your sexual health?

Chapter 12

Recreational Health:
Feeding the Soul with Fun

The right use of leisure is no doubt a harder problem than the right use of our working hours. ~~ Dean Inge

Fun feeds the soul, and without it our inner light will die. Though the serious nature of the human condition lends itself to much distress and heartache, the joy of the soul—its essence—is the light that reminds us that we are alive. It is also the light that guides us to soul health and can guide us through our entire experience of the human condition, if we allow it.

The more advanced a society becomes, the less pure fun and joy we seem to have in our lives. Too often, we use our leisure time for sports and other forms of competition instead of for activities that produce simple laughter and joy. We more often look for joy outside ourselves than ever in human history.

This chapter explores the recreational branch of health, which is best served by our innermost sources of joy and laughter and depends also on how we define ourselves by our leisure time. The recreational branch is the most overlooked when we consider health in general; however, even minimal attention to this branch enhances our well-being and soul health.

Joyful Soul

Death is not the greatest loss in life. The greatest loss is what dies inside us while we live. ~~ Norman Cousins

I have long lost track of how many people have entered my psychotherapy office bringing with them their sorrows, but leaving behind any sense of joy. They have lost their enjoyment and feel as if their zest for life has completely disappeared. When asked, few can say what used to make them smile, let alone remember the last time they really laughed. When I ask what they do for fun, the all-too-common answer is "nothing." Certainly, when people are anxious, depressed, grief-stricken, stressed, or in any other state of turmoil, their experiences of joy are rare. But reacquainting with what brings them joy is guaranteed to free them from the gravity of any challenging circumstance or situation.

Our soul is *nothing* without joy. Without joy we are void of all light that reminds us why we live. In times when the human condition has us in its darkened grip, our experience of joy is less tangible, and so is our connection with our soul. We cannot see as clearly how to make decisions that suit our wisest ally, and we often go further off track rather than closer to our inner wisdom. Consequently, it's not unusual for people who are distressed to report that they no longer know who they are, as their despair further disconnects them from their soul.

Our sense if joy—or lack of one—, thus, serves as another measure of our soul health. Our sense of joy is much like the pilot light for our inner ally—as long as it is lit we are still experiencing at least some pleasure in life and are able to tolerate the darker sides of the human condition. However, when that light is dim or snuffed out, nothing seems to matter—not even oneself. Therefore, awareness of what brings us joy is of utmost importance to our overall health. Essayist Logan Smith notes, "If you are losing your leisure, look out; you may be losing your soul." Indeed, our souls do define us; and if we don't listen to them, we will never find our way back home to this inner ally. More tragic is the risk of losing who we really are.

Joy stems both from the fun and leisure we create in our lives and from the meaning we place on the activities we choose for recreation. Individual recreational needs may differ as widely as the people on the planet do. What we all have in common, though, is that fun and leisure not only buffers the unpleasant aspects of our human condition, but also fortifies or feeds the soul.

The recreational branch of soul health relates to both the fun *and* the leisure we allow, invite, or create in our lives. There is a difference between the two, though. We experience fun through "acting playfully"—reacting in a light-hearted, humorous, or jesting manner —at home, work, or social situations. Leisure time, however, allows us to find respite from our responsibilities—personal and professional—which usually represent the heavier aspects of our human condition. Both fun and leisure are necessary in fortifying our soul and promoting its evolution.

Unfortunately, most people don't make or take time for fun and leisure. In a 2010 survey, an online travel agency found that only 38 percent of Americans use all of the vacation time they were allotted. This may not be surprising, given the standards for long hours of work in this country; however, the physical and emotional cost may outweigh the praise we get for the long hours worked. In fact, there is often a direct impact on physical health when people don't take time to relax. One researcher found that people who don't take time to slow down from daily life may find it harder to relax in the future since the neural pathways that produce feelings of calm and peacefulness become weaker, making it increasingly more difficult to shift to less stressful states of being. This demonstrates that our bodies are indeed restored when we are at rest or at play—and that this is necessary in sustaining our well-being.

Research also shows that people who don't take time off for vacations are at higher risk for serious health conditions and also shortened life spans. The Framingham Heart Study, likely the most comprehensive ongoing research on the development of heart disease, has followed twelve thousand men for over a decade to see if there are ways to improve both health and longevity. The study found that people who took frequent breaks or vacations from work tended to live longer. A survey done in the state of New York indicated that men who took annual vacations reduced their risk of death by 20 percent, while those who had taken no vacation within the preceding five years had the highest incidence of heart disease than any other men surveyed.

The positive impact of leisure time is unquestionably good for mental as well as physical health. A study of women who took frequent vacations showed that they were less likely to become depressed, anxious, or fatigued, and they also reported less stress at home.

Overall, leisure time consistently shows positive enhancement of health. Not only does time away from everyday stressors allow us to reconnect with ourselves, but there is clear evidence that intentionally planning leisure time into our lives promotes creativity, staves off burnout, recharges our batteries (both physically and mentally), promotes overall well-being, improves higher performance and productivity once back at work, and strengthens the bonds between people outside of work.

Fun—our ability to let loose and play— is highly under-rated among adults. As our responsibilities increase, our pursuit of fun decreases, often drastically. And the longer we go without this pleasure, the less we seem to think it is a priority. Even so, how many people do you know who fantasize over working more versus playing more? It seems that even when we wish for more fun and time to play, we often don't make a point of creating this in our lives.

Biologically speaking, fun does more than soothe the soul. When we engage in playful activities, our serotonin level—the substance balanced by a typical antidepressant—boosts instantaneously. In addition, our stress hormones drop, our endorphins—the natural pain killers—increase, and sometimes adrenaline rises, too, which boosts our energy levels. If that isn't enough proof that fun is good for our health, then consider that vicarious enjoyment—just watching others play or laugh—is also enough to boost these chemicals.

Laughing at *yourself* also helps with managing difficult experiences within the human condition. This self-directed joviality has been shown to lighten our perception of stressful events and allows us to maintain a level of resilience in the midst of life's battles. We cannot deny the issues that need work in life, but the research does offer hope for a healthier life when we can think of the events of everyday life as manageable. In other words, when we find humor in the human condition, we can heal many aspects of our soul health.

Despite the positive effect of pure fun and leisure, many people nevertheless either avoid them or think they are unworthy of joy or unable to experience it. Unfortunately, they often turn to unhealthy substitutes such as alcohol, other drugs, over-spending, sex, gambling, or any other vice that may temporarily numb their stress. The problem with these substitutes is that they always negatively affect other branches of soul health. These substitutes for joy further disconnect people from their soul, often while actively damaging the health of other branches. This can create a vicious cycle; they dig themselves further into the ditch of ill soul health, only to continue seeking false relief through one of their vices.

The ability to recognize that your recreational branch of health needs work takes honesty and courage, given that the work may go against what you were taught a child. If your caregivers were workaholics, overachievers, or simply naysayers about fun, your sense of self-worth may influence you to follow in their footsteps. If your parents weren't playful or fun, you may not have learned to integrate it into your own life. But, no matter what the reason, if you don't feel you have enough fun and leisure in your life, you probably don't.

Below is the Questionnaire for the Recreational Branch of Health. Take some time to evaluate your own ideas of fun and leisure as well as how they have affected your soul health.

QUESTIONNAIRE FOR THE RECREATIONAL BRANCH OF HEALTH

On a scale of 1 to 10, rate the level of your health within each area described. A 10 describes optimal, radiant health, while a 1 describes an almost complete lack of health within the given aspect of the recreational branch. Remember, this questionnaire is designed to create a roadmap to overall radiant health. It is not meant to overwhelm you.

Fun

1. _____ I have enough fun in my life.
2. _____ I know what is fun to me.
3. _____ I take time to have fun.
4. _____ I laugh often.
5. _____ I play often.
6. _____ I am playful with others.
7. _____ Others think I am fun.

Leisure

1. _____ I know how to relax.
2. _____ I have enough leisure time.
3. _____ I actively seek time to relax.
4. _____ I plan ahead for time away from work.
5. _____ I use all vacation time that is allotted to me.
6. _____ I use my weekends to relax.
7. _____ I engage in healthy activities that put me at ease.
8. _____ Leisure time is a high priority for me.

Balance

1. _____ I maintain a good balance between work and leisure.
2. _____ I actively work to create and maintain balance in my life.
3. _____ I rarely feel physically or emotionally drained.
4. _____ Most people would say I have a well balanced life.
5. _____ I know when to take a break from busy or stressful activities.
6. _____ I plan ahead for busy or stressful times when I know I will need leisure time.

Beliefs about Fun and Leisure

1. _____ Fun and leisure are important to me.
2. _____ I know it is okay to have fun.
3. _____ I know it is okay for others to have fun.
4. _____ I know it is okay to need and take time to rest.
5. _____ I am comfortable with having fun.
6. _____ I am comfortable with having down time or leisure.
7. _____ I know that fun and leisure are important for overall health.

Outlook on Life

1. _____ I can laugh at myself.
2. _____ I try not to take life too seriously.
3. _____ I look for ways to see the bright side in life.
4. _____ I stop to notice the things happening around me that are fun and entertaining.
5. _____ I can find joy in even the little things.

Like the other branches of soul health, the recreational branch consists of many elements that you might never have considered. Your ability to recognize the differences among fun, leisure, and life balance, to understand your beliefs about them, and to identify your general outlook on life all help you feed your soul. Most importantly, your willingness to create a strong recreational branch can fortify and boost your resilience in handling more stressful or challenging aspects of the human condition.

FUN

What soap is to the body, laughter is to the soul. ~~ Yiddish Proverb

The word "fun" means "to behave playfully." And when we do so, it clearly does our soul good. There is nothing better for your soul than an uncontrollable belly laugh that brings you to the point of tears and leaves your sides aching, your energy spent. No other experience feeds your soul more than these hearty bouts of mirth and no other experience leaves your soul more content.

One study shows that the average four year-old laughs three to four hundred times a day, while adults average fewer than four times a day. When I share these statistics in workshops, a sad, desperate sigh usually fills the room and most agree that they do not have enough fun or laughter in their lives.

No matter how you look at it, fun is under-rated. Research is clear that laughter, itself, produces multiple health benefits including a decrease in blood pressure and stress hormones, an increase in endorphins (natural pain killers) and immunity to illness, and fewer physical effects of stress altogether. Thus, if you have a lot of fun in your life, you can bet that you will be healthier than those who have lost their joy and therefore have more emotional and physical ailments. Not only does the fun in your life heal your body, it also soothes your soul.

> » When was the last time you behaved playfully rather than acted for a purpose other than fun?

> » What fun are you leaving out of your life?

> » Are you resentful of others who seem to have more fun than you?

> » Have you forgotten what makes you laugh?

LEISURE

He enjoys true leisure who has time to improve his soul's estate. ~~ Thoreau, Henry David

Relaxation has become a lost art. Few people know how to create ease in their day and find respite from the everyday grind. In our world the hustle and bustle of life is valued far more than relaxation, despite the often desperate voice of the soul asking them to slow down. In fact, it often takes the demand of illness to make them rest.

What's interesting is that most people long for the time to slow down—they hear the voice of their soul longing for a break—yet they never take the time to actually do it. Only by putting some distance between themselves and their responsibilities can they gain the break they need from the human condition, find a new perspective, and organize their lives in such a way that they don't return to the same exhausted and overwhelmed existence.

Research shows repeatedly that problem-solving, clarity of thought, creativity, efficiency, and even hopefulness about stressful situations all increase after time spent away through vacations or even short, deliberate periods of leisure. The biggest obstacle to this healthy kind of action is the willingness to give oneself permission to slow down and relax. If only people would understand that leisure necessary not just to survive the human condition, but also to thrive within it.

» What do you do to relax?

» Do you do these things often enough?

» What sort of leisure do you long for but not allow yourself to have?

» What obstacles do you place between yourself and your leisure?

» Do you give yourself permission to rest or relax when you need to?

BALANCE

To the art of working well a civilized race would add the art of playing well. ~~ George Santayana

Soul health is all about creating life balance so that you can reach your most optimal way of living. But few people factor recreation into their pursuit of health, despite how much they may long for more fun and leisure in their lives.

The truth is fun and leisure can be found in each and every other branch of health. Still, for many people, seeking recreational health can feel like work because, like all other branches, it requires a conscious process. But once they identify their key ingredients to this branch of health—their fun factors and most effective forms of relaxation—all they have to do, in order to satisfy the soul, is make and an ongoing commitment to engage in those activities. Most people enjoy very simple pleasures—what feels like work is taking the time to engage in them.

Your balance will not find you; you must find it. Creating your own equilibrium in life can, itself, be fun if you let it. Many clients have left my office enjoying the thought that their assignment for the week was to have more fun, and they returned feeling at least some sense of renewal and liberation from their daily stress.

» How do you know when you are out of balance?

» What do you do when you become aware of imbalance?

» What is your plan to reclaim balance in your life?

BELIEFS ABOUT FUN AND LEISURE

All of us, from time to time, need a plunge into freedom and novelty, after which routine and discipline will seem delightful by contrast. ~~André Maurois

We are a product of our environment. And if your upbringing instilled a lack of balance in your beliefs about work and play, you probably brought this into adulthood. Though it is admirable to have a strong work ethic, this alone won't feed your soul. And it certainly won't grant you permission to laugh and play nearly as often as your soul health might require.

In our culture, it is not uncommon for people to feel guilty when they have fun or take time to relax, and this often keeps them from doing so. Somehow, they have accepted the idea that such pursuits are self-indulgent, despite how much better they feel when they engage in them. This may have nothing to do with money, and instead have everything to do with the idea that they don't deserve the time or energy it takes have fun or relax.

Because the recreational branch of health is key to understanding and experiencing radiant living, it is important to look at fun and leisure as an investment in soul health. Rarely does anyone get to the end of life and wish they had worked more; instead, most wish they had spent more time engaging in fun or leisure. Their regret inevitably diminishes their soul health.

» What are your beliefs about work and play?

» Do they match your ideas about radiant health?

» Do you feel guilty when you engage in fun and leisure activities?

» What fun and leisure activities would you regret denying yourself in the next week? The next month? Year? Lifetime?

OUTLOOK ON LIFE

Laughing gives divine perspective. ~~ Alison Stormwolf

The way you look at life is how you will experience it. If you are a glass-half-empty person you will experience a half-empty life, always coming up short of what you wish you had done. However, if you see things from a brighter perspective, you are likely to have more joyful options than you know what do to with. Remember—the soul has simple needs. It is our human condition that complicates our outlook on life.

Certainly, for the sake of soul health we must take life seriously, but the ability to laugh at ourselves in the midst of our trials and tribulations is essential as we search for a healthier and more balanced life. Life always feels lighter when we meet it with a positive or even joyful attitude, looking for opportunities to grow in any given situation. In essence, joy is the fertilizer of our soul—it helps to both buffer and to enhance our human condition and fosters our inherent ability to expand our overall consciousness.

If joy is the fertilizer of the soul, then laughter is the detergent—it clears away the debris left by struggle and pain and sharpens the inner eye to see the potential beyond the hard times. In our challenging, overly busy times, we tend to get so locked into the messiness of life that we can't gain enough perspective to see the humor in it. Lightening up can provide a welcome respite from the serious or troublesome aspects our human condition.

> » In what part(s) of life do you need to lighten up?

> » How easily do you find the humor in your own situation?

> » What can you do to see your life as more full rather than empty of joy?

THE PLAYGROUND OF THE SOUL

To share laughter is to connect with Soul. ~~ Alison Stormwolf

Play is a great way to connect with others. Laughing and having fun not only helps us to bond more deeply with other people, but also to enter a deeper understanding and connection with our own soul. Laughter unlocks our resistance and releases inhibitions, thus opening us to close connections that might not arise without this mutual joy.

The soul craves connection. It wants to be understood, heard, and embraced by those who can appreciate and honor it—oneself, especially, but close family and friends as well. Only then can the soul itself play. It wants the freedom to revel in whatever elicits its joy, experiencing every aspect of fun and elation that life has to offer. However, as we all know, there are times when life could not offer less fun. Those are the times when a playful connection with our own soul and others' is most distant, yet most vital.

Just like any playground, the human condition can create bumps and bruises amidst the fun and laughter. Yet even in the worst of times, it is often our ability to see the humor in our situation that allows us to muddle through it. Finding joy in the midst of darkness allows us to soften the impact of life's challenges and open us to the possibilities that something good could come from our pain. The key is to understand yourself well enough to know when you need a good dose of fun, or when laughter will be your own best medicine.

EXERCISE

What is fun to you? Stop right now and list ten things that you do or could do on a regular basis that would be *fun*. How difficult is it to create this list? Who do you have the most fun with in your life? How often do you spend time with these people? Who would you invite into your personal playground if you could?

What *relaxes* you? Stop and list ten leisure activities that you do on a regular basis. How difficult is it to create this list? Who do you relax with the most? How often do you take time to relax with those who make it easy for you to do so?

Answering these questions will help you to create your soul's playground. By identifying what and who helps you strengthen your recreational branch of health, and by committing to doing what enhances it, you will give your soul reason to sing. You will also enhance its evolution.

No one can deny that they feel the most radiant and alive when they have had a good dose of pure fun. Our driven culture often dismisses and even denies how important simple joy is to our health, yet the lack of it drives many of our vices and unhealthy behaviors. The reality is, if we tuned into our inner joy more often—regardless of our daily struggles— our soul health would be much brighter. Instead, we keep losing sight of the inner light and are frantically searching for other ways to soothe our discomfort.

What do you need in order to commit to joy?

PART TWO

SOUL-BASED LIVING

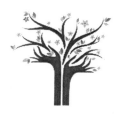

*The personal life deeply lived always expands
into truths beyond itself.* ~~ *Anais Nin*

CHAPTER 13

YOUR TREE OF LIFE:
ALIGNING WITH SPIRIT

By this point in the book, you have already evolved somewhat within each branch of the Soul Health Model. Your awareness has grown—your knowledge of who you are and what you do and do not need to reach your optimal health in each of the ten key components of the human condition. Your inner voice is stirring—and likely telling you more about what you need to clean out or fill up in order to live life more radiantly. You are never finished evolving, though no one is. Now is the time to connect the dots more completely.

This chapter will help you work in tandem with your soul on a minute-to-minute basis. Your progress will show you your unique path to soul health. I emphasize "unique" because, despite what others or society may tell you, soul health is a completely individual experience—only *your* soul knows what *you* need to feel radiant.

THE TREE OF LIFE

The meaning of life is not to be discovered only after death in some hidden, mysterious realm; on the contrary, it can be found by eating the succulent fruit of the Tree of Life and by living in the here and now as fully and creatively as we can. ~~ Paul Kurtz

The Tree of Life symbol has long been used in science, philosophy, religion, mythology and various spiritual contexts to illustrate unity and connection among all living things. In the case of the Soul Health Model, however, your tree belongs entirely to you because your overall health is completely in your hands.

This is *your* life, *your* soul, *your* health, *your* path, and *your* journey. In other words, your tree will differ from others' and that it is to be embraced and celebrated as you learn to work more closely with your inner life source—your soul.

As mentioned throughout the preceding chapters, your inner wisdom—the voice of your soul—operates constantly in order to guide you. It is the force that draws you toward people, things, and experiences that feed your willingness to live and urges you to fight for life at all cost. It is also the force that attempts to guide us away from the people, things, and experiences that may harm us. Your soul creates your sense of well-being—or alerts you to the lack of it—as it guides you along your path. Most importantly, your soul is what assists you in your unique path of evolution, helping you live more radiantly instead of succumbing to the hazards of the human condition.

The Soul Health Model provides the blueprint to your essential needs for the ten key branches of your health. From the purely human side of our experience, these branches must be repeatedly balanced and attended if you seek whole health. But it is the *alignment* with your soul—a deep connection with your inner ally that will allow you to experience the genuine soul health—for which everyone yearns.

ALIGNING WITH YOUR MOST VITAL ALLY

To attain inner peace you must actually give your life, not just your possessions. When you at last give your life—bringing into alignment your beliefs and the way you live, then, and only then, can you begin to find inner peace. ~~ Peace Pilgrim

Aligning with your soul means getting to know it and learning to work in tandem with it to create the most optimal and radiant life you could imagine. Much like entering a new friendship or other relationship, you must get to know yourself at the deepest level in order to truly experience soul health. This has probably become obvious as you've worked your way through each chapter so far. As you learn to understand yourself better in each branch of human health, you inevitably come to understand yourself more deeply at the soul level as well. Building knowledge and awareness about yourself in regard to each branch, provides the roadmap to balance and enhance your personal tree of life. Although this roadmap may change a bit from time to time throughout your life, the components that are most important to you will likely remain fairly stable. They are your core needs—the nutrients—that your soul requires in order to thrive. Working to fulfill these core needs will guarantee not only radiant health, but also your soul's evolution. Your growth is as simple as that.

It is impossible to separate our complicated daily lives from our soul. When the human condition is making us feel bad, our soul aches, too. We become unsettled, unhappy, and anxious and long for some sort of change, something that will soothe our *dis*-ease,—something that will soothe our soul. Once we are calmed, the angst of our inner voice subsides and we return to a more contented satisfaction with life. However, if we don't attend to our discontent, it can fester into any kind of ailment that afflicts mind, body or spirit. If, instead, we forge a working alliance between our human condition and our soul, our *dis*-ease can be amazingly short-lived and we can maintain a state of whole health.

Things arranged in tandem are "one behind the other." We might say, then, that our soul is behind us all the way. Even if we aren't aware of it, or familiar with it (being out of touch with ourselves), it is constantly backing us up, trying to get our attention and help us find our highest good—our soul health. But many of us aren't very astute about these inner stirrings. Few have been trained or have discovered that this inner ally is our best defense against the hardships of the human condition. The soul knows all the twists and turns that our lives can take, and it has the solutions for every one of them. We just need to align with the soul —tune in and pay attention—to understand its supportive guidance more clearly.

This is where consciousness comes in. Earlier chapters mention that radical consciousness is essential to understanding ourselves, our condition, and our soul's evolution. As we become more aware of the whole picture, we can work more effectively with the soul to create our best possible experience on this planet. That seems to be what we all want but don't know how to achieve. The Soul Health Model allows you to consciously examine each branch of your life in order to not only to live more fully, but also to collaborate with your soul to create your optimal health.

Partnering with our soul is the only way the tree of life can flourish—it is the only way we will thrive and the only way our souls will evolve. When the ten key branches of our tree are cared for and healthy, they are aligned with our soul's absolute truth, which sets the stage for our evolution. This alignment gives us our most accurate awareness of who we are so that we can act with precision in fulfilling our soul's needs. Our absolute truth *IS* our radiance—it is the wisdom that lights our path to evolution. Our radical consciousness of this is the key to radiant living.

THE FOREST VS. THE TREES

You have to leave the city of your comfort and go into the wilderness of your intuition. What you'll discover will be wonderful. What you'll discover is yourself. ~~ Alan Alda

Over seven billion human beings occupy this planet, all of them with their own trees of life, complete with their own soul health, whether is it optimal or suffering in some way. With this in mind, it is no surprise that it can be extremely difficult to create your own soul health while others' agendas can get in the way or inhibit your evolution.

Our primary mission, both as humans and as souls, is to get to know ourselves at the deepest possible level. But this is hard, and it is scary. We encounter myriad difficult events—accidents, illnesses, challenges, tragedies, divorces, births, and deaths—, and all of them can derail us from our alignment with our soul. We can also experience many wonderful events such as healthy relationships, births, adventures, and achievements. All are universal aspects of the human condition that many would prefer not to experience—for better or for worse. Nevertheless, I am absolutely convinced that our most difficult challenge is knowing ourselves at the soul level. It can be more difficult and more scary because it requires us to turn the mirror on ourselves, look at what is not working in our lives, and accept who we are and who we have become so that we can identify what we need to change to align with our inner ally.

While doing so, it can be tedious to figure out what is our own stuff and what is others'—what is our responsibility to work on or change and what is another's—, particularly if we accept life at face value and have little clear knowledge about human dynamics. People are complicated, which means that both we and others can complicate life. Our lives are challenged both by what we learn from others, and also by whatever dramas we create for ourselves. We can be sure that the soul is not "behind" many of these detours; instead, it is the many facets of the human condition that provides the lessons from which to learn and allow our souls to evolve.

On the other hand, our soul *is* behind the discomfort that makes us want and need to get out of distress. It is trying, through its discomfort, to tell us that we're on the wrong path—that we must re-align in order to regain the contented state of equilibrium. In a rather ironic way, our soul causes our emotions, aches, and pains to flare in its attempt to get our attention and prompt us to right something that has gone wrong. If we ignore it, our situation will get worse, compounding our *dis*-ease until we finally listen. In some unfortunate cases, these messages are ignored to the point that the soul itself goes dormant until something comes along to re-awaken it. With this in mind, the human condition—which might feel more like the dark and malevolent forest—must be separated from your tree of life before you can see the way out.

Take, for instance, a woman who continues to find herself in abusive relationships. At first, each relationship seems new and fresh, with her partner paying great attention to her and making her feel like a queen—or at least like someone cares. After a while, the forest begins to darken. Her partner becomes less attentive and more demanding. His original charm has turned to a confusing mix of manipulation, deceit, and possessiveness. Somehow she's led to believe he is jealous and protective of the relationship just because he cares so much. He apologizes and says he will never mistreat her again. Life feels sunny once more, as he says that he will change. Then, the emotional confusion returns, this time with verbal accusations, name calling, and even an occasional threat or show of violence. The darkness of the forest deepens until, once more, he shifts and swears that he will stop. The woman believes him—because she wants to. And because she has seen him be attentive and possessive in the past—all of which is because he loves her so much. As the forest continues to darken, she moves further into the woods, to the point where she cannot recognize her own tree among the oppressive vines and leaves. Her light is too dim for her to distinguish herself from the forest. Her soul is immobilized and she is stuck, cycling through the endless promises and disappointments.

Although this example may seem extreme and dramatic to some, it is not uncommon. It is also not the only forest waiting for the unaware. Others may include the limitations of our parents' or caregivers' beliefs and behaviors, the influences of our peers and teachers during our school years, the friendships and partnerships we form along the way, societal beliefs, values, and norms of our culture—whether they pertain to gender, ethnicity, politics, race, or religion—, factors in our work environments, and more. Given the complexity of the world around us, it is a wonder that anyone can think or feel for themselves, let alone discover and honor their soul.

The human condition is our forest and our soul is our very own tree. Those who come to *know* themselves can align more directly with their soul. The victory of life is to be able to live through your soul, not through or for the other trees or the forest.

Consciousness can be described as your emergence from the woods or dark forest. You were born into this world as a soul within a human body and it wasn't until the human condition pulled you in that you entered the forest and perhaps even got lost there. The forest is the land that is unfamiliar and distant from your soul.

Soul health is all about this awakening—this deepening of a connection that will never allow you to lose sight of your inner light again. It is your emergence from the dark woods—the expectations, norms, peer pressures, and other constraints—that allows you to reconnect with your soul and commit to leaving the forest behind, living through your soul and entering your own realm of conscious evolution.

LIVING THROUGH THE SOUL

*Every man dies—Not every man really
lives.* ~~ William Ross Wallace

As both a human being and a soul, it is your right to discover, honor, claim, and live in constant communication with your soul. Yes, the human condition, or forest around you, can make it difficult and even impossible at times to do so. But it is still your right and your ultimate choice. Following are the steps to living through your soul and thus paving the path to your radiant health:

1. Listen within.

    Throughout this book you have been encouraged to listen to the voice within in order to hear what you really want and need—or don't—in order to experience deeper satisfaction with life. Along the way, you have encountered several examples, exercises, and suggestions for doing these things. If you have found it difficult to hear your inner voice, I would suggest seeking help from a therapist or other professional. Note, though, that not all professionals are trained for this kind of work and it is important for you to receive guidance that will help *you* and not the "forest" around you.

2. *Hear* the message.

    Often, in our humanness, we miss multiple cues from our soul which may have been trying to guide us all our lives. We have not been trained to listen for the inner voice, and in many cases we may have been cautioned or even chastised for doing so. Listening to oneself above others—particularly for women—has been punished and dismissed as selfish or unimportant. But remember that discovering and partnering with the soul is our human right. Hearing the messages from within tells us that there is meaning behind our *dis*-ease. We wouldn't be ill at ease unless our soul was trying to say something. Learn to listen to your emotions, your aches and pains, and any thoughts that are too insistent to ignore. Your soul is sending messages it wants you to hear through these signals. It wants you to evolve beyond whatever is creating the *dis*-ease.

3. Interpret the message.

Though we have not been trained to seek deeper meaning to our *dis*-ease, there is *always* a meaning behind anything and everything that makes us less than content. Our discontent is what indicates that we are not aligned with our soul. Learn your own soul language. Notice the patterns for when your discontent or your aches and pains arise. Pay attention to how, when, and why your emotions get triggered. And, again, seek assistance if you feel you are missing the point of an inner message. Sometimes our human condition blurs or muffles an alert from our soul, so the help of an objective voice such as a therapist or other guide—though intimidating at first—can show you how to interpret your soul's message.

4. Separate your tree from the forest around it.

Find ways to distinguish your thoughts from others', your feelings from those of the people around you, and your ideas and beliefs from those that prevail in the world at large. Figure out what is yours from what is theirs and strengthen your ability to root yourself in an understanding of what your soul wants and needs in order to survive and thrive. Recognize that your soul is yours and yours alone. If you do not listen to it and honor it, no one else will— or can.

5.   Prioritize your soul.

Many believe it is selfish to live through the soul, acting on their own needs and beliefs. But there is a huge difference between being selfish and living *for self*. Selfish people are chiefly devoted to or concerned only with themselves and their desires. In other words, they have an agenda that disregards others and have little or no concern for them or their needs. Soul health is entirely different. In fact, it is impossible to be selfish—that is, to not consider others—if we are truly living through our soul, because when we act through the purity of our inner wisdom, our actions work for the alignment and purity of all others as well. For instance, when we assert ourselves with others, for the sake of our soul health and not our ego, arrogance, or greed—factors of the human condition—, we educate another's soul; we demonstrate how to rise above self-interest alone. Saying yes to what another person wants when you know it will work against your soul health will only dishonor your own soul—*and* the soul of the other person, whether they realize it or not. You may not give the person what they want, but it may very likely be what they need. Selfishness is often perceived by those who are selfish themselves. Actions that serve the soul, on the other hand,—those that are *for self* rather than *selfish*—will be well-received by those who likewise honor their souls and aren't caught in the pitfalls of the human condition.

Prioritizing your soul is of utmost importance in creating

radiant health. Without this vital step, you might as well go back into the forest.

6.   Commit to your conscious evolution.

Evolution is the gradual process of changing into a new and better form. In serving soul health, your commitment to consciously evolve is essential. If you leave your tree as it is you will never feel better. Your tree will never enter new levels of growth or development, you most certainly won't feel free of your discontent or *dis*-ease, and more importantly, you won't evolve. As long as you choose not to grow or learn, the distressing aspects of the human condition will continue to loom and haunt you. You will remain in your dark forest, without an awareness of your inner self. Your soul will be lost beneath the human condition and you will feel as if you are merely existing and not truly living. Choosing to live through your soul—to understand the dimensions of soul health and to work toward soul alignment—is the only path to evolution. The choice is up to you, as is the result.

By now, of course, you understand that when you commit to soul health you commit to evolve. For instance, the woman in that abusive relationship would—whether she realized it or not— be committing to her evolution if she recognized how unhealthy the relationship was and decided to leave it. If she avoided the temptation to return, or to get into another damaging relationship, that would confirm her evolution beyond her previous level of soul health. In other words, any time you work to improve and steadily maintain your soul health, you are also acting upon the choice to evolve.

Thus your own tree of life and your soul health are synonymous. Finding radiant living is only a matter of determining what you need at the soul level and executing a plan to reach it. Yes, it's a process and yes it can be difficult or challenging. But what feels worse? Evolving—or choosing not to? Regret is the side-effect of refusing to evolve. The problem is the resulting scars or knots in our tree stay visible throughout our lives. They are reminders of the detours we took on our path to our soul's evolution.

It's time to choose your soul health—to choose evolution. How ready are you?

CHAPTER 14

SOUL HEALTH PLAN:
TAKING ACTION FOR RADIANT LIVING

You can live a lifetime and, at the end of it, know more about other people than you know about yourself. ~~ Beryl Markham

We are often so busy attending to others that we don't know how to care for our own soul. By now, though, you are more aware of how you can reach a more optimal level of living.

This chapter will help you to assimilate more fully everything you have learned about yourself from the individual chapters on soul health. If you follow the five steps listed below, you will be able to create a formal soul plan for assessing and envisioning your radiant living.

SOUL STEPS TOWARD RADIANT LIVING

Step 1

The questionnaires included in Chapters 3 through 12 have helped you get a better idea about what needs attention in each of the ten branches of your soul health. Below, you will find a Soul Health Assessment that you are to respond to directly from your inner wisdom, which provides the viewpoint of your soul. When you assess each branch from a soul-based level you will achieve a deeper understanding of your unique soul needs.

The Soul Health Assessment will yield a numerical result that will show you which branches need attention, and which ones are most urgent to address. As you consider each statement, give it a rating from 1 (almost never) to 5 (almost always). The branches with the lowest total scores are the ones you need to work on first—they are the most in need of your attention.

Remember—evaluating your branches of soul health should not overwhelm you, but simply guide you on your path to radiant health. For that reason, no generalized numerical measure of ideal radiant health is necessary, since you cannot compare your unique tree of life to any other. The numerical ranking system is simply a guide to a relatively objective understanding of where to start on your Soul Health Plan. The next chapter offers greater detail on how to make a plan for soul health.

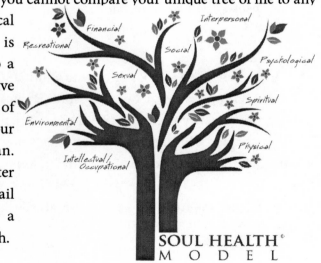

Financial

Interpersonal

Recreational

Social

Psychological

Sexual

Spiritual

Environmental

Physical

Intellectual/
Occupational

SOUL HEALTH
M O D E L

SOUL HEALTH ASSESSMENT

PHYSICAL HEALTH

1 2 3 4 5   I know that physical health is important to my overall soul health.

1 2 3 4 5   My soul feels healthy, vibrant, and strong.

1 2 3 4 5   I understand what my soul tells me about my body.

1 2 3 4 5   I know how to care for my body at the soul level.

1 2 3 4 5   My physical health shows that I take good care of my soul.

1 2 3 4 5   My soul is happy with how I treat my body.

1 2 3 4 5   My soul informs me about my nutritional needs.

1 2 3 4 5   I eat only what creates a healthy body and a healthy soul.

1 2 3 4 5   My soul is satisfied with my level of physical activity.

1 2 3 4 5   My levels of sleep and rest reflect a healthy soul.

1 2 3 4 5   I understand that ailments are often symptoms of an uneasy soul.

– – – – –

Total: _____

PSYCHOLOGICAL HEALTH

1 2 3 4 5   My soul feels at ease.

1 2 3 4 5   My soul tells me what I need to change in my emotional life.

1 2 3 4 5   My soul is reflected in my positive thoughts about myself.

1 2 3 4 5   I know and accept who I am at the soul level.

1 2 3 4 5   My soul is open to joy and love.

1 2 3 4 5   My emotional boundaries align with the needs of my soul.

1 2 3 4 5   I allow the world to see who I am at the soul level.

1 2 3 4 5   My soul knows I take good care of my psychological health.

1 2 3 4 5   I am deeply at peace with myself.

1 2 3 4 5   I know my emotions are messages from my soul.

1 2 3 4 5   My soul is satisfied with where I am in my life.

— — — — —

Total: _____

Social Health

1 2 3 4 5   I have enough social support to satisfy my soul.

1 2 3 4 5   I have only soulful relationships with others.

1 2 3 4 5   I recognize when a relationship is unhealthy for my soul.

1 2 3 4 5   My family is supportive of me at the soul level.

1 2 3 4 5   My friends are supportive of me at the soul level.

1 2 3 4 5   The people in my life are good for my soul.

1 2 3 4 5   My soul is satisfied with the time I spend with others.

1 2 3 4 5   My soul is filled rather than depleted by the people in my life.

1 2 3 4 5   My soul is at ease with the people in my life.

1 2 3 4 5   My soul is at ease in most social situations.

1 2 3 4 5   My life is filled with people who are healthy for my soul.

— — — — —

Total: _____

INTERPERSONAL HEALTH

1 2 3 4 5   My soul is satisfied with the kinds of relationships I have.

1 2 3 4 5   My soul is satisfied with how others treat me.

1 2 3 4 5   The people in my life respect me at the soul level.

1 2 3 4 5   I communicate what I need from others to honor my soul.

1 2 3 4 5   I actively resolve conflict so that my soul can be at ease.

1 2 3 4 5   My soul is safe with the people in my life.

1 2 3 4 5   The needs of my soul are honored by others in my life.

1 2 3 4 5   My relationships reflect the needs of my soul.

1 2 3 4 5   The people in my life understand me at the soul level.

1 2 3 4 5   My soul alerts me when others place conditions on our relationship.

1 2 3 4 5   I leave relationships that are not healthy for my soul.

– – – – –

Total: _____

INTELLECTUAL/OCCUPATIONAL HEALTH

1 2 3 4 5   My soul is satisfied by my occupational/intellectual efforts.

1 2 3 4 5   I only pursue intellectual challenges that are right for my soul.

1 2 3 4 5   I solve occupational problems based on what my soul needs.

1 2 3 4 5   My soul is challenged, not bored, by my life overall.

1 2 3 4 5   My work feeds my soul.

1 2 3 4 5   My work is aligned with what I truly want in life.

1 2 3 4 5   My outlook is generally positive.

1 2 3 4 5   I see intellectual challenges as opportunities for my soul to grow.

1 2 3 4 5   My soul embraces change rather than fears it.

1 2 3 4 5   My soul tells me when to take a break from intellectual work.

1 2 3 4 5   I know that my outlook on life affects the health of my soul.

— — — — —

Total: _____

Environmental Health

1 2 3 4 5   My home environment reflects the needs of my soul.

1 2 3 4 5   I know that my personal choices affect the world around me.

1 2 3 4 5   My soul feels connected to the natural environment.

1 2 3 4 5   My respect for the earth is reflected in my actions.

1 2 3 4 5   I actively create a personal environment that supports inner peace.

1 2 3 4 5   My belongings help me to feel at peace.

1 2 3 4 5   I honor the earth as I would my own soul.

1 2 3 4 5   I know that my personal environment mirrors the health of my soul.

1 2 3 4 5   My soul feels at ease in my home environment.

1 2 3 4 5   My soul feels at ease in my work environment.

1 2 3 4 5   My environment reflects my core beliefs.

— — — — —

Total: _____

FINANCIAL HEALTH

1 2 3 4 5   I am at peace with my current financial situation.

1 2 3 4 5   I am at peace with how I spend money.

1 2 3 4 5   I make financial decisions based on what my soul needs.

1 2 3 4 5   My soul is comfortable with how I save money.

1 2 3 4 5   My purchases are more need-based than frivolous.

1 2 3 4 5   I feel grounded when I make most purchases.

1 2 3 4 5   My soul is at ease with my level of debt.

1 2 3 4 5   My soul is at ease with my financial future.

1 2 3 4 5   I know when a purchase feels wrong to my soul.

1 2 3 4 5   My soul is at ease when I think about money.

1 2 3 4 5   My soul knows I take care of my finances.

– – – – –

Total: _____

SPIRITUAL HEALTH

1 2 3 4 5   I look for the deeper meanings of events in my life.

1 2 3 4 5   I actively practice my spirituality.

1 2 3 4 5   My soul is at peace with my spiritual beliefs and practices.

1 2 3 4 5   My spirituality fills my soul.

1 2 3 4 5   My soul tells me when it needs spiritual attention.

1 2 3 4 5   I can share my spiritual beliefs with the people in my life.

1 2 3 4 5   My spirituality is important to the health of my soul.

1 2 3 4 5   I actively seek spiritual activities to in order to grow.

1 2 3 4 5   I know that my spirituality helps my soul to evolve.

1 2 3 4 5   Quiet time helps me hear my soul more clearly.

1 2 3 4 5   I know what my soul needs to feel spiritually satisfied.

– – – – –

Total: _____

Sexual Health

1 2 3 4 5   My sex life satisfies my soul.

1 2 3 4 5   I am at peace with my sexuality.

1 2 3 4 5   I only engage in soulful sex.

1 2 3 4 5   I am at peace with my sexual interests and needs.

1 2 3 4 5   I only engage in sex with soulful partners.

1 2 3 4 5   I am at ease with my sexual past.

1 2 3 4 5   My soul feels safe when I engage in sex.

1 2 3 4 5   I am able to enjoy sex.

1 2 3 4 5   My soul feels at ease when I think about sex.

1 2 3 4 5   I know that soulful sex requires a mutual decision.

1 2 3 4 5   After having sex, I never feel my soul has been dishonored.

– – – – –

Total: _____

Recreational Health

1 2 3 4 5   My life is filled with joyful activities.

1 2 3 4 5   My soul is satisfied with the fun in my life.

1 2 3 4 5   My soul is satisfied with the leisure in my life.

1 2 3 4 5   I would describe my soul as joyful.

1 2 3 4 5   I actively create fun to feed my soul.

1 2 3 4 5   I actively create leisure to restore my soul.

1 2 3 4 5   My soul tells me when I need more fun and leisure in life.

1 2 3 4 5   I know what is fun to me.

1 2 3 4 5   I know what restores my soul.

1 2 3 4 5   My soul is at peace with what I do for fun.

1 2 3 4 5   I know that fun and leisure are important to soul health.

–   –   –   –   –

Total: _____

Step 2

Now that you have completed the Soul Health Assessment, list below the three branches of soul health that had the lowest scores in ascending order:

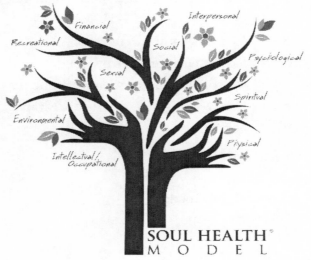

1)   (lowest score)   _____

2)   (next lowest score)   _____

3)   (third lowest score)   _____

Take a minute to decide if these are the branches that you feel need the most attention or whether others feel like higher priorities given your current situation. If you need to reorganize your branches, do so, since your soul may be guiding you to the areas in most urgent need of help. Your gut (soul) reaction will tell you whether you have prioritized these appropriately.

Step 3

Before you go on to create your Soul Health Plan, it is important to have a clear vision of what you want to achieve. I encourage you to find a quiet, uninterrupted time to envision how you want your soul health to be in one year. Try to envision how you want your life to look and feel in each of the branches of soul health as well as how you would after reaching this level of radiant living. Spend some time exploring every detail you can imagine at this level of radiance.

Now take some time to write down this vision to include:

1. How your soul health would feel in one year.

2. What would be different about *you* as a result.

3. What would be different about your life.

4. How much more life or radiance you would experience.

5. How much more fulfilled you would be.

Take as much time as necessary exploring your thoughts about your vision of soul health. The clearer and more detailed your vision, the more easily you will achieve it. Of course, be realistic about what you can achieve in a year, but stick to your vision so you don't lose sight of what you are truly striving for.

SOUL HEALTH PLAN

Step 4

This is where you begin to improve your health on each of the branches you identified as being in need of work. Keep in mind that when one improves, the others will also shift in a more positive direction. The interrelationship among the branches is synergistic: that is, the effect of working on individual branches affects the whole system. So, although you will create a plan to work on each separate branch, you will positively affect the other branches and your entire tree of life.

In the process, you will more specifically identify within each branch: 1) what needs to be cleaned out or eliminated, and 2) what needs to be filled up or fortified. Remember that it is often necessary to make room for positive growth by removing obstacles that block the way to soul health. Be as honest and specific with yourself as you can, using your soul to guide you. Keep in mind, we only achieve what we can indentify specifically, so avoid generalized answers and allow your soul to guide you in the work that needs to be done to enhance your tree of life. Use a journal, notebook, or the spaces in this book to complete the following outline:

PRIORITY BRANCH # 1 _____

What needs to be *eliminated* from this branch of soul health?

1. _____

2. _____

3. _____

4. _____

What steps must *you* take to clean out this branch?

1. _____

2. _____

3. _____

4. _____

What needs to be *fortified or filled up* in this branch of soul health?

1. _____

2. _____

3. _____

4. _____

What steps must *you* take place in order to fill up this branch?

1. _____

2. _____

3. _____

4. _____

PRIORITY BRANCH # 2_____

What needs to be *eliminated* from this branch of soul health?

1. _____

2. _____

3. _____

4. _____

What steps must *you* take place in order to clean out this branch?

1. _____

2. _____

3. _____

4. _____

What needs to be *fortified or filled up* in this branch of soul health?

1. _____

2. _____

3. _____

4. _____

What steps must *you* take place in order to fill up this branch?

1. _____

2. _____

3. _____

4. _____

PRIORITY BRANCH # 3_____

What needs to be *eliminated* from this branch of soul health?

1. _____

2. _____

3. _____

4. _____

What steps must *you* take place in order to clean out this branch?

1. _____

2. _____

3. _____

4. _____

What needs to be *fortified or filled up* in this branch of soul health?

1. _____

2. _____

3. _____

4. _____

What steps must *you* take place in order to fill up this branch?

1. _____

2. _____

3. _____

4. _____

Step 5

Now that you have completed this process, you have identified at least some steps you need to take to create a more fulfilling level of soul health. However, because you are human, you will probably hesitate to follow through with some of the actions identified above. To evolve beyond any blockages, ask yourself the following questions (and remember it is useful to write your responses down as you go, because this will help you reach a deeper soul level):

» What obstacles do I see in following through with any actions I need to take?

» What will it take for me to remain conscious of my goals?

» How do I sabotage my own growth and evolution?

» What would I regret more—growing or not growing?

» What assistance do I need in my process of reaching optimal soul health?

» How willing am I to seek and make use of this help?

» What needs to happen before I can follow through and honor my soul?

Our human condition—the basis of our fears and flaws—is always a factor when we try to change something in our lives. Unexpected shifts in our lives also affect our ability to follow through with our plans. But the greatest roadblock to soul health is within you. Once you overcome your mental and emotional roadblocks, you can find radiant health.

Step 6

Getting out of your own way is, therefore, the most important part of reaching soul health, even though it is often the most difficult part of it as well. However, setting your personal soul health plan also takes considerable self-awareness, including a strong sense of what most reliably helps you to succeed.

Now that you have completed the first five steps, it is time to set some goals for your one- year mark. Keep in mind that evolution is a process and that it takes conscious effort on your part. This is the only way to create and maintain your path to soul health.

Consider the following:

» Do you do better with daily, weekly, or monthly goals?

» Do you need someone or something to keep you accountable?

» How do you best monitor your progress (even if you don't like doing it)?

» How will you know if you are getting off track?

» How will you know when you need help to reach your goals?

Step 6 entails actually setting your goals and getting to work on them. This part is entirely in your hands, since only you know your soul. Your gut—or soul—will know how to help you set your goals, if you allow it. Consider the following method of identifying your goals:

1. What does your gut (soul) say about setting goals for soul health?

2. How will your soul tell you when you aren't working for its benefit?

3. What sort of gut (soul) reaction will tell you when you are off track?

Take some time now to plan whatever feels right to you in your commitment to achieve your vision of soul health in one year. Trust that your soul knows best, and allow it to guide you as you write down what your path to soul health will entail. Write this down so that you can revisit it at any time. You may often need to remind yourself what your soul wants. Living and acting through the soul takes listening to it and following its instructions. You know this from everything you have read in this book, and yet it is easy to lose sight of.

I encourage weekly exploration of your progress since this is helpful in assessing whether you are moving in the direction of soul health. I have also found that it is helpful to review your progress made every two or three months, because the longer time shows you that you are actually achieving goals along your path to optimal health. Taking the time to stamp or affirm your progress is a necessary part of growth and it also helps you decide on the next step you need to take toward evolution.

Once you have completed the steps in this chapter, you are likely to keep on creating your ultimate soul health. The next chapter emphasizes the importance of becoming a steward of your soul as you proceed.

CHAPTER 15

SOUL STEWARDSHIP:
TENDING YOUR SOUL'S GARDEN

Every spirit builds itself a house, and beyond its house, a
world, and beyond its world, a heaven. Know then that
world exists for you. ~~ Ralph Waldo Emerson

Originally, stewards were household servants chosen by their
master or lord to attend to every need—bringing them food
or drink, arranging social occasions, dressing them in the morning,
and running every detail of the estate. Today, stewardship can also
refer to our personal responsibility to manage everything in our
lives. Our conscious evolution requires us to manage more than the
nourishment of our body and conduct of everyday lives; we also have
the ultimate responsibility for the health of our soul.

This chapter explores and emphasizes the need to adopt an
ongoing, proactive stance on soul maintenance. Without a conscious
understanding of our soul-based needs, as well as what can get us
off track from meeting them, our soul health is jeopardized and our
evolution is thwarted. Discernment—the ability to identify the needs

unique to our individual soul health—is key in becoming a good steward to your most vital ally.

DISCERNMENT

Re-examine all that you have been told...dismiss that
which insults your soul. ~~ Walt Whitman

Discernment is an acquired skill, one that is necessary in becoming a good steward to your soul. Those who learn to discern their soul's needs are able to sense when something is amiss and what needs to be done to correct it. Developing this skill may require you to remove something from your life that is obstructing optimal health or add something to it that can fortify your soul. Once you become aware of what your soul needs, it is up to you to provide it.

Becoming a good steward of your soul means attending consciously to its needs at all times, regardless of your circumstances, and remaining in a constant state of *conscious evolution*. This is the soul's most desired and natural state. True stewardship of our soul requires not only a commitment to listen and respond to its inspiration, it also means being willing to act upon what we learn through our discernment process, even if the steps do not seem logical.

For instance, in completing the Brief Soul Survey in Chapter 1, you took a quick glance at the ten key branches of health necessary to create the conditions for your soul's evolution. Through consciously exploring the branches, you were likely "discerning" as you recognized that soul health has many more facets than you might originally have thought. Then in later chapters, as you completed the questionnaire for each branch of soul health, your consciousness about what healthy branches require became clearer. Later, as you completed the Soul Health Assessment in Chapter 15, you were asked to consider more deeply the factors that not only affect the health of each branch, but your soul health as a whole. Each step of the assessment raised your awareness of what you needed to do at each branch to fulfill your own optimal health and thereby your soul's unique needs. This process also provided insight into how each branch interacts with and affects the others. The more you know about what you need, the more discerning you can be in creating your radiant health.

While discernment is an internal, proactive process, stewardship to your soul requires external action. It relies entirely on your willingness to execute the change that will stimulate your soul's evolution and maintain your healthy balance in the human condition. This is a challenge for many, even those who have a good understanding of spiritual concepts. But one must remember that no matter how much knowledge you hold about spirituality, evolution does not truly occur until we, as humans, take the right actions.

The core emphasis of the Soul Health Model is the understanding that as we create the best possible balance of all aspects within the human condition—the branches of our tree of life—we also set the stage for our soul's evolution. Without this attentiveness to our various human needs, we neglect the soul as well—and vice versa. It is imperative to understand that our stewardship of our souls requires us not only to function well as humans, if we wish to evolve beyond our situations, but also to rely on our spiritual nature to facilitate the process.

I often ask clients whether they want to heal their wounds or evolve beyond them. Often, the question puzzles them because they never considered the difference. However, once clients explore their options, they inevitably choose the acts that lead to evolution. Stewardship of our souls requires not only the ongoing awareness of our needs, but also the willingness to support and even sustain our soul's evolution at all costs. Because our souls are here to evolve, true stewards of their soul will accept whatever challenges the human condition presents in order for them to grow, however difficult they may be.

For example, most of my clients eventually come to the point in therapy where it is much more uncomfortable to remain mired in their human condition than to forge ahead and make the changes necessary for them to grow. This is a conscious action, a result of knowing what they need to do to change—spiritual discernment—, followed by their stewardship of their soul in actually doing something to change their situation. One cannot be a soul steward without developing an awareness of what it needs in order to grow. Discernment and a commitment to active soul stewardship create the only avenue to the soul's pure and unimpeded evolution.

EXERCISE

Take some time now to consider whether you have been a good steward of your soul. Explore the ways you have or have not honored your soul, and consider what happened as a result.

We inherently know when the deepest part of us is pleased with how our life is going because we feel content or settled. Stewardship of the soul creates satisfaction that nothing else can emulate. Our soul knows when our human life is aligned through stewardship, because that is when we feel the most at peace with our actions and choices, regardless of how difficult it may have been to decide on the actions that bring us to that point. Any form of discontent means we have some work to do to rebalance our lives and thus become better stewards to our soul. Practice becoming more aware of your inner peace to determine how good of a steward you are to your soul; this will ensure not only our inner peace, but also your soul's evolution.

YOUR SOUL'S GARDEN

Let us be grateful to people who make us happy, they are the charming gardeners who make our souls blossom ~~ Marcel Proust

One way to become a better steward of your soul is to envision your tree of life as its own garden. The Soul Health Model provides a kind of landscape from which to work, and your job is to practice ongoing discernment about its condition and its needs. Every garden goes through seasons of growth, and every healthy garden requires regular attention in order to thrive.

When I bought my house it needed a lot of work—both inside and out. I tend to like making my house my own, so this wasn't an obstacle for me. But I had no idea what sort of evolution would take place right in my own front yard.

My house sits back from the street behind a small hill that partially obscures the front of it. No one from the road gets to see what I do from my front porch, and at the time of purchase I was glad they didn't. Looking out my front door you see the side of the hill that is not visible from the street. When I moved in, this area was completely covered in vines and weeds. I knew there was a stone wall somewhere along the bottom of the hill, but I had no idea what else I would find once I unburied the stone barrier.

It took me nearly three months to completely clear away the unruly vegetation. But in doing so, I slowly realized the treasure that was hidden beneath. Once cleared, the slope facing my house turned out to be a terraced garden with three levels of stone walls alternating with bushes, shrubs, and plants that I couldn't see at first. However, an even more amazing evolution occurred throughout the year following my mass cleaning project. New to the region, I was unfamiliar with native plants; however, slowly but surely, new plants started popping up, stretching up through their newly cleared space and presenting themselves in a huge variety of shapes and colors. The poor things had had no room to grow in their vine-covered prison and no way for the sun to touch them and bring out inherent beauty. All along, I was tending an unseen garden that had been long neglected, and I was rewarded with multitudes of beautiful buried treasures. To this day, I cannot believe that someone allowed these riches to become buried.

Our souls are much like this garden, and we must consciously and constantly tend them. The process is as simple as cleaning out what has died away in our lives, or doesn't feed us any longer, and filling up, or replacing them with what nourishes or fertilizes our optimal health. This process takes time. Just as we experience many different cycles in life, the seasons of our soul present many opportunities to refine our lives to our radiant living.

The seasons of the soul are much like those in tending a garden. There are times for preparing the ground, planting seeds, waiting for germination, nourishing and weeding the plot (maintenance), harvesting flowers or fruits, and settling the garden for winter (rest). These all compare to phases we cycle through many times in our lives. Becoming conscious of these cycles allows us to embrace them more fully and act on behalf of our soul.

Preparation Phase—People in the preparation phase may either feel stuck or unproductive or be starting to make the necessary shifts they need to in order to set new behaviors or thoughts into motion. This is often a time of incubating ideas and energy rather than actually changing routines or patterns, though it can feel frustrating nonetheless. Because growth and change always feels better than being stuck, this stage often creates an anxious anticipation of something that may be just around the corner, yet still out of sight. This is also a time when people assess aspects of their life that need change—such as the branches of the Soul Health Model. This stage may include weeding out things that no longer fit in their lives, redesigning their ideal tree of life, and identifying what needs to be planted or shifted for the landscape of the soul to finally take shape.

Planting Phase—This stage marks the beginning of actual, outwards changes. As I tell clients in my therapy office, people don't tend to change unless they are tired enough of their situations or themselves. So, the planting phase marks the end of feeling "stuck" and the beginning of new growth. Although the changes may still feel preliminary, they are of utmost importance to the development and deepening of discernment. They lead to a new awareness of what to plant for the sake of the soul, and what to leave behind that may have been obstacles to radiant health. Setting goals, taking positive steps toward growth, and intentionally implementing change in one's life are all part of the planting phase.

Germination Phase—Seedlings take time to sprout. Our growth toward soul health can feel slow at first, but through conscious exploration and action we can make the changes necessary for a stronger, more radiant life. Patience, perseverance, and commitment are necessary at this key point in your evolutionary process, especially because it is when many people revert to old ways, finding it too hard or too time consuming to generate new habits or beliefs. Some may believe the payoff in growth is not large enough for the amount of work that goes into it, or they may feel they don't have the time, patience, or courage to wait for the signs of growth to appear. But once growth is apparent, even in the most vulnerable, early stages, it is well worth the wait. The soul pays dividends when it has what it needs to grow. An inner sense of forward movement is all it takes for people to realize that their hard work is paying off. The job at this point is to maintain the process long enough for new growth to mature.

Maintenance Phase— Maintaining growth can be a struggle. Because we are steeped in the human condition, our old habits sneak up and try to lure us back to our old ways. Either that or unexpected events in life will throw us off track, pulling us away from our best intentions and back into our old routines. Maintaining the soul's garden requires us to continually monitor our growth, weed out any persistent, unhealthy thoughts or behaviors that try to creep in, and nourish ourselves through life-affirming activities. This determination yields a soul-deep sense of relief as new habits are created and new ways of living happen more naturally. The challenge, though, is to maintain this momentum until our efforts for growth and change come to fruition.

Harvest Phase—People know they have entered this phase when they can reap the benefits of their hard work and change. This is when they feel they are filling up or repairing a part of their soul that they previously neglected. In this phase, as their garden matures, life is richer and more fulfilled. Those who have maintained their commitment to growth begin to feel pride in the results, and this spurs more areas of growth.

Rest Phase— The soul never stops its influence on our lives, though it does need time to pull back from our efforts to reflect.

Although few people know how to actually listen to their inner ally, it is constantly active, either in trying to get our attention through physical, emotional, spiritual or other cues, or in helping us make decisions based on our gut—our soul-based instincts. However, there are times when we must reflect on our human condition long enough to take stock of our current level of growth and plan for the next one.

Stewardship of the soul is an unending process—it involves many overlapping and ongoing cycles throughout our lives, and it requires a conscious commitment. If we neglect stewardship, our lives become overgrown or stagnant in one way or another, and this makes it harder to connect with our soul.

» What can you do to be a better steward of your soul?

» What would help you remain conscious of what needs work from day to day?

Given the complexity of the human condition, good stewardship of the soul requires periodic reevaluation of every branch of soul health. As life ebbs and flows, each branch shifts priority depending on its condition. Some branches just seem to even out without much help, while others may need more attention as they weather life's storms. When this happens, I would suggest reviewing the Soul Health Survey and/or the individual assessments found in the chapter that focuses on the branch in question. However, for those who are ready to commit to a daily commitment, consider using the following questions as a daily measure of soul health.

GUIDE TO DAILY SOUL HEALTH

Use the following questions for daily devotion to your Soul.

How has my soul thrived today?

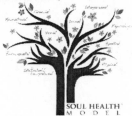

How has my soul struggled today?

Which branch or branches needed the most attention today?

What did I do today to rebalance this branch (or these branches)?

What can I do tomorrow to enhance my soul health?

What can I do tomorrow that will prevent an imbalance of my soul health the next day?

SOUL MISSION

In order to reach optimal radiant health, you must honor your commitment to your soul. One way to do this is to create a personal Soul Mission Statement of your intention to act as a good steward. Your soul is your primary audience for this mission statement, so it is important to be very clear about what you write and say.

A mission statement is a timeless definition of a)who you are, b) of what your main purpose in life is, c) of your core values, d) of your reason for existence, and e) of your mission, or task you aim to fulfill. It may seem odd to write a mission statement to your soul, but the act of creating one is another exercise in knowing your own soul ever more deeply. In carefully and consciously crafting your statement, you come to know exactly what you are striving for and whom you are serving at all times; it is the ultimate commitment to your soul.

My own mission statement reads as follows:

I am a vehicle of consciousness whose mission is to elevate others to reach radiant health and ultimate soul evolution. I strive to educate others to thrive in life while also serving as an ongoing role model in seeking and maintaining my own optimal soul health. I see life as a healing journey, one which is available to all souls, most of all one's own, but one which is always subject to the curiosities and challenges of the human condition. I am committed to my own soul health, growth, and evolution both for myself and for the souls that I am fortunate enough to serve.

Although the first sentence of this mission statement sums up my love of helping others, it is the commitment to my soul that allows me to do this. Once you recognize what your mission statement is, it shapes your entire tree of life in service of soul health. Finding your mission in life often takes time, but in many cases you are already fulfilling this mission, you just don't know it.

Take some time now to develop your Soul Mission Statement,

based on what you know of yourself at this point, after working on your soul health. Keep in mind that although mission statements are meant to be timeless, you will likely change and refine yours as you get to know yourself and your soul. This is a lifelong process, but keeping your statement in mind will help you balance the branches of your tree of life and stay aligned with your soul health.

Stewardship to your soul is a never-ending process. Although it takes time to reach radiant soul health, daily soul stewardship is what allows you to get there. By committing to your soul, you are ensuring your growth and evolution. Your Soul Mission Statement will set the stage for doing this throughout your life.

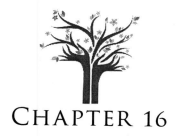

CHAPTER 16

SUMMARY:
MAINTAINING THE PATH TO RADIANT LIVING

*Our own inner intelligence is far superior to any we can try
to substitute from the outside.* ~~ Deepak Chopra, M.D.

S taying on the path to soul health takes only the commitment
to do so. Our inner wisdom allows us to reach radiant living
if we let it, which means it is up to us to learn how to listen to our
inner voice and master aspects of our human condition. Declaring
your commitment to your soul is the most vital pledge you will ever
make. Without it, you are likely both to struggle to make sense of
your everyday life and to inhibit your evolution beyond it.

VIRTUES OF CONSCIOUS EVOLUTION

By now you surely realize that soul health is a process, not a
destination. We are never finished evolving and although we need
periods of rest and reflection, we must always sustain conscious
balance in our lives in order to grow. Although we are human beings

having a spiritual experience, we often forget the spiritual part and stay stuck in being human. We will stumble over and over again on our path to wholeness, but as long as we pick ourselves back up and continue onward, we will remain on our path to evolution. We can use many human tools or virtues in the process of tending our soul's garden:

Honesty— "To thine own self be true." Our soul health is unattainable without self-honesty. The Soul Health Model represents all aspects of the human condition that we must be aware of and be addressing before we can reach soul health. Our willingness to be honest about what we need and don't need for the health of every branch in our tree of life sets the stage for our growth.

Courage —Change takes courage. Old habits, patterns, ideas, and beliefs are hard to break, and letting go of them takes a heightened awareness. We may experience many forms of trauma, drama, and tragedy in our lives—as part of our human condition—, but facing ourselves and learning our lessons is the hardest thing we can ever choose.

Commitment —Change takes courage and evolution takes commitment. Because soul health is a process, paying unfailing attention to our inner ally requires a life-long commitment. However, I've found that once people learn to grow they never want to stop. Movement is always more fulfilling than stagnation.

Diligence—Staying on top of your growth is an ongoing challenge, but when you adopt a stance of radical consciousness, your soul rewards you many times over. This keeps the process going—your hard work brings returns, which motivates more hard work. The payoff— constant growth— is exponentially greater than the effort required for action.

Perseverance—Enduring "the good, the bad and the ugly" of the human condition is easier when we keep a steady focus on our goal, which is radiant living. Our willingness to push through the tough times—those that are usually the most fertile for growth—allows us to persevere regardless of the challenges or obstacles before us.

Creativity—Surviving the human condition takes determination; thriving within it requires creativity. Our soul can provide magnificent creative resources when we seek it and the wonderful part is that creativity itself is inevitably fulfilling.

Patience— "Love is patient, love is kind." Even the oldest souls can worry that their periods of growth take a great deal of time. Like fine wine, we often must age in order to gain inner wisdom. Being patient with ourselves and our experience of the human condition is often the biggest challenge to our evolution.

Self-Love—Though it may sound like a cliché, you really must love yourself in order to love others or the life you have been given. And to experience radiant living, you must fall in love with your soul. You must honor and cherish it in the way you would your most adored other person. But few people do open their hearts to their soul, not realizing that this is the largest obstacle to receiving what they want the most—love and inner peace, which is the same thing as optimal soul health.

Compassion— As human beings, we are certain to fall flat on our faces, humiliate ourselves, and make seemingly fatal mistakes in our lives. Having compassion toward ourselves at these times may be difficult, but it soothes the soul in a way that nothing else can. Nurturing ourselves through our mistakes or fumbles allows us to move beyond them more quickly and enter a state conducive to our soul's evolution.

Humor—Last, but certainly not least, is to see humor as a genuine virtue in dealing with our daily struggles. It is, perhaps, the most important of all our tools to be able to laugh at ourselves and our situations. When we can be amused by our own foibles, we can avoid being victims. Laughter dislodges us from the human condition and elevates us above our challenges. Adopting a comical perspective will broaden your view of life beyond what embarrassment, judgment, or fear will allow.

UNTIL WE MEET AGAIN

I recently talked with a colleague about this book and its purpose—to help others reach their optimal level of radiant living and thus pave the way for soul evolution. She asked me where I thought we were evolving to—and I quickly replied "To oneness". The truth is, the more we align with our souls the more we also align with other people—with other souls. In finding our deepest and brightest inner peace, we learn to express and share what everyone desires— a contented harmony that begins in our depths and radiates outward to others. This light converges to create a greater sense of connection with every other soul—oneness between all that exists. Nothing can feel wrong or disconnected in this state of being, because the troubles and fears of the human condition can no longer have a negative impact on us—we can rise above the human condition and evolve beyond it, simply observing ourselves in our everyday lives instead of becoming absorbed by our daily challenges.

With this in mind, know that I am with you on your journey—and so more than seven billion others on this planet. Know that the human condition is just that—a condition—something we can all evolve beyond. Know that we are all in this together, experiencing, learning, growing, and evolving. Know that the human condition is something to be embraced, observed, laughed at, and risen above. Know that your soul longs for you and can't wait to become reacquainted. Most of all, know that the radiant living that comes from soul health is yours if you want it. Your soul awaits you.

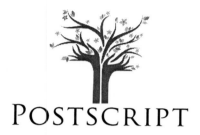

POSTSCRIPT

Our experience on earth is about more than just surviving the human condition; it is about mastering it. I am aware that soul health is a new concept, one that is foreign to many. Expanding our conceptualization of health deepens our understanding of our daily struggles and their impact on overall health, as well as assists us in becoming more conscious of the ultimate reason we live—to evolve our souls.

Many are concerned with the current state of our healthcare system. My concerns are many. Our souls have gotten lost amid managed healthcare, the Medicare Part D coverage gap (a.k.a. the "Medicare donut hole"), much of medical research and technology, the general separation between mind, body, and spirit in our treatment of symptoms, the lack of education (for both the public and healthcare professionals) concerning all of the aspects—or branches—of human life that affect health, and the disjointed nature of medical care as it has evolved—or devolved—to a "specialist" approach rather than an integrated or holistic one. In the current system, there is no such thing as "whole health." It is now up to the individual to reacquaint oneself with the entirety of who we are and to learn to view our soul as an asset on the road to true health.

During this time of expanding consciousness, it is imperative that we come to understand our role in the advancement of the human race. Our evolution is dependent on our willingness and ability to recognize how the health of our soul will help us not only thrive as individuals, but also reunite as a collective society. When we lose the soul of the individual, we lose the soul of the human race. We become disconnected from everything and everyone around us, and chaos ensues in one way or another. Many would argue that we've already lost the collective soul, but as in the human condition, even the earth's population as a whole must undergo its challenges in order to "re-correct" and grow individually, as well as become a unified whole.

The events of the last decade have offered endless opportunities to expand our consciousness about how we live as humans and also to connect—or reconnect—with those around us. The worldwide financial crisis has shown many that it is time to scale back and live within our means. Corporate restructuring is forcing many workers to take a closer look at whether they are happy in their jobs, careers, and work environments, and has inspired many to pursue their life's passion or calling. The overturning of many governments indicates a readiness for egalitarian leadership—a coming together into a more cohesive group through acceptance of differences, rather than the pulling apart of society which occurs with judgment. The countless natural disasters—earthquakes, tsunamis, tornados, floods, avalanches, hurricanes, volcanic eruptions, blizzards, dust storms, and more—offer lessons of gratitude, preparedness, humanitarianism, and altruism as well as an awareness and acceptance that the planet really is in trouble. Gas shortages, food contamination, epidemics, abuse scandals, divisive presidential campaigns and elections, mass shootings, terrorist attacks, and so much more are fertile ground for awareness and growth beyond what is accepted at face value. There is greater meaning behind each event if only we would allow our awareness to expand. All of these events, disasters, and scandals are messengers of consciousness; we just need to more deeply read the memos.

Consciousness, itself, is not a new concept. But many continue to focus on what is happening right before them rather than expand their view to recognize how everyone and everything is connected. Victor Frankl, Anne Frank, and Helen Keller are just a few historic examples of people who have shared their observations of the human condition despite their challenging—and even horrific— circumstances, and embraced a much bigger picture of their purpose and lessons on earth. More recently, Steve Jobs, Apple Computer's late co-founder, was able to view his life to extract its meaning and present the 2005 Commencement Address that created a viral explosion of internet viewings. Malala, the 14 year-old Pakistani girl who spoke out about the injustice of restricting women in their culture from receiving an education, showed the world through her relentless courage that even an assassination attempt would not stop her from returning to school.

Our collective consciousness expands every time a person shares a new awareness about their lives with another. Our evolution to "oneness" is the ultimate level of soul evolution. But we have a long way to go before we get there. The truth remains, there is much to learn from the human condition; and consciousness is the teacher.

Everything that affects our life also affects our soul. And everything we learn as a result of life expands our consciousness. Although radiant health may seem out of reach to many, I have witnessed countless examples of clients and others who have done their work and reaped the benefits of a balanced and vibrant life. Light, itself, can move both around and through objects. Similarly, as humans, we can feel the essence of the soul brighten despite the trials and tribulations of daily life if we choose to learn from our difficult experiences. It is through the inspiration of our soul that we glow and, ultimately, grow.

It's time to choose consciousness. It's time to evolve.

REFERENCES AND SUGGESTED READING

Abbey, Antonia, Zawacki, Tina, Buck, Philip O., Clinton, Monique, and Mcauslan, Pamet. 2001. "Alcohol and Sexual Assault." *Alcohol Research and Health* 25 (1): 43-51.

Abram, David. 1996. *The Spell of the Sensuous: Perception and Language in a More-Than Human World.* New York: Pantheon Books.

American Psychiatric Association. 2000. *Diagnostic and Statistical Manual of Mental Disorders DSM-IV-TR (Text Revision).* Arlington, Virginia.

Athanasiaus of Alexandria. 1892. "On the Incarnation of the Word." In *Nicene and Post-Nicene Fathers,* edited by Philip Schaff. New York: The Christian Literature Company.

Ban Breathnach, Sarah. 1995. *Simple Abundance: A Daybook of Comfort and Joy.* NewYork: Grand Central Publishing.

Barker, Phil & Buchanan-Barker, Poppy. 2005. *Breakthrough: Spirituality and Mental Health*. London: Whurr Books.

Barral, Jean-Pierre. 2007. *Understanding the Messages of Your Body: How to Interpret Physical and Emotional Signals to Achieve Optimal Health*. Berkeley: North Atlantic Books.

Beinfield, Harriet. & Korngold, Efrem. 1991. *Between Heaven and Earth: A Guide to Chinese Medicine*. New York: Ballantine Wellspring/Random House Publishing Group.

Bennett, M.P. & Lengacher, C. 2008. "Humor and Laughter May Influence Health: Laughter and Health Outcomes." *Evidence-Based Complementary and Alternative Medicine* 3 (1): 61-63.

Bennett, M.P., Celler, J.M., Rosenberg, & McCann, J. 2003. "The Effect of Mirthful Laughter on Stress and Natural Killer Cell Activity." *Alternative Therapies in Health and Medicine* 9 (2): 38-45.

Blanchflower, David G. & Oswald, Andrew J. 2004. "Money, Sex, and Happiness: An Empirical Study." Cambridge, MA: National Bureau of Economic Research.

Bonierbale, M, Lancon, C., & Tignol, J. 2003. "The ELIXER study: Evaluation of Sexual Dysfunction in 4557 Depressed Patients in France." *Current Medical Research Opinion* 19 (2): 1114-1124.

Bureau of Labor Statistics. 2011. "2011 American Time Use Survey Summary." Accessed November 2012. http://www.bls.gov/nls/nlsfaqs.htm#anch43 .

Carbon Footprint. 2012. "The Carbon Footprint." Accessed November 2012. http://www.carbonfootprint.com .

Chase, Steven. 2011. *Nature as a Spiritual Practice*. Grand Rapids, Michigan: Wm. B. Eerdmans Publishing Company.

Chikani, V., Reding, D., Gunderson, P., & McCarty, C.A. 2005. "Vacations Improve Mental Health Among Rural Women." *Wisconsin Medical Journal* 104 (6): 38-44.

Craigie, F. 2010. *Positive Spirituality in Health Care*. Minneapolis, MN: Mill City Press.

Culliford, L. 2002. "Spiritual Care and Psychiatric Treatment: An Introduction." *Advances in Psychiatric Treatment* 8: 249-261.

Dalai Lama. 2009. *The Art of Happiness: A Handbook for Living*. New York: Riverhead Books.

De Chardin, Pierre Teilard & Appleton-Weber, Sarah. 1999. *The Human Phenomenon*. Eastbourne, United Kingdom: Sussex Academic Press.

Dossey, L. 1989. *Recovering the Soul: A Scientific and Spiritual Search*. New York: Bantam Books.

Dossey, L. 1995. *Healing Words: The Power of Prayer and the Practice of Medicine*. San Francisco: Harper San Francisco.

Dossey, L. 1999. *Reinventing Medicine: Beyond Mind-Body to a New Era of Healing*. San Francisco: Harper San Francisco.

Eisenstein, Charles. 2011. *Sacred Economics: Money, Gift & Society in the Age of Transition*. Berkeley, California: Evolver Editions.

Englehart, Matthew & Englehart, Terces. 2008. *Sacred Commerce: Business as a Path of Awakening*. Berkeley, California: North Atlantic Books.

Expedia.com. 2011. "Deprivation Study." Accessed April 2012. http://www.expedia.com.

Framingham Heart Study. 2007. Accessed April 2012. http://www.framinghamheartstudy.com

Hay, Louise. 1984. *You Can Heal Your Life*. New York: Hay House.

Hettler, Bill. 1977. *The Six Dimensions of Wellness Model*. Chicago: National Wellness Institute.

House, Freeman. 1999. *Totem Salmon: Life Lessons from Another Species*. Boston: Beacon Press.

Jaksch, Mary. 2011. *Start Over: Create the Life YOU Want*. Seattle, Washington: Amazon Digital Services. Kindle Edition.

Jawer, Michael A. & Micozzi, Marc S. 2009. The Spiritual Anatomy of Emotion: How Feelings Link the Brain, the Body, and the Sixth Sense. Rochester, Vermont: Park Street Press.

John-Roger & Kay, Paul. 2010. *Living the Spiritual Principles of Health and Well-Being*. Los Angeles, California: Mandeville Press.

Karpinski, G. 199). *Where Two Worlds Touch: Spiritual Rites of Passage*. New York: Ballantine Books.

Koenig, Harold G. 1999. "The Healing Power of Faith." *Annals of Long-Term Care* 7 (10): 381-384.

Koenig, Harold G. 2008. *Medicine, Religion, and Health: Where Science and Spirituality Meet*. West Conshohocken, PA: Templeton Foundation Press.

Koenig, H., McCullough, M. & Larson, D. 2001. Handbook of Religion and Health. Oxford: Oxford University Press.

Kovescses, Zoltan. 2003. *Metaphor and Emotion: Language, Culture, and Body in Human Feeling (Studies in Emotion and Social Interaction).* New York: Cambridge University Press.

Lang, Frieder R. & Fingerman, Karen L. 2009. *Growing Together: Personal Relationships Across the Life Span.* New York: Cambridge University Press.

Laumann, Edward et al. 2006. "A Cross-National Study of Subjective Sexual Well-Being Among Older Women and Men: Findings from the Global Study of Sexual Attitudes and Behaviors." *Archives of Sexual Behavior* 35 (2): 143-159.

Levin, J. 2001. *God, Faith and Health: Exploring the Spirituality-Healing Connection.* New York: John Wiley and Sons.

Lincoln, M. 2006. *Healer's Handbook for Practitioners: Messages from the Body, Condensed Version.* California: Talking Hearts.

Maltz, Wendy. 2012. *The Sexual Healing Journey: A Guide for Survivors of Sexual Abuse.* New York: Harper Collins.

Margolis, C. 2008. *Discover Your Inner Wisdom: Using Intuition, Logic, and Common Sense to Make Your Best Choices.* New York: Fireside Books.

Maxwell, John. 2004. *The Journey from Success to Significance.* Nashville, Tennessee: Thomas Nelson, Inc.

McLaren, Karla. 2010. *The Language of Emotions: What your Feelings Are Trying to Tell You.* Boulder: Sounds True.

Merton, Thomas. 1961. *New Seeds of Contemplation.* New York: New Directions.

Myss, Carolyn. 2001. *Anatomy of the Spirit.* Boulder: Sounds True.

National Humane Society. 2011. Accessed March 2012. http://www. humansociety.org.

Noelle, Scott. 2008. *The Daily Groove: Parenting…Unconditionally!* Portland, Oregon: Create Space.

Oelschlaeger, Max. 1994. *Caring for Creation: An Ecumenical Approach to the Environmental Crisis.* New Haven: Yale University Press.

Pert, Candace. 1997. Molecules of Emotion: The Science Behind Mind-Body Medicine. New York, New York: Simon and Schuster.

Piff, P.K., Stancato, D.M., Cote, S., Mendoza-Denton, R., & Keltner, D. 2012. "Higher Social Class Predicts Increased Unethical Behavior." *Proceedings of the National Academy of Sciences of the United States* 109 (11): 4086-4091.

Pilates, Joseph H. 1998. *Your Health: A Corrective System of Exercising that Revolutionizes the Entire Field of Physical Education.* Ashland, Ohio: Presentation Dynamics/Atlas Books.

Plotkin, Bill. 2008. *Nature and the Human Soul: Cultivating Wholeness and Community in a Fragmented World.* Novato, California: New World Library.

Post, S. & Puchalski, C. M. 2000. "Physicians and Patient Spirituality: Professional Boundaries, Competency, and Ethics." *Annals of Internal Medicine* 132: 578-583.

Puchalski, Christina M. 2001. "The Role of Spirituality in Health Care." *Baylor University Medical Center Proceedings* 14: 352-357.

Puchalski, C. & Ferrell, B. 2010. *Making Healthcare Whole: Integrating Spirituality into Patient Care.* West Conshohocken, PA: Templeton Press.

Randall-Young, G. 2004. *Growing into Soul: The Next Step in Human Evolution.* Victoria: Canada: Trafford Publishing.

Rath, J. 2007. *Strength Finders.* New York: Gallup Press.

Rawlins, William K. 1992. *Friendship Matters: Communication, Dialectics, and the Life Course (Communication & Social Order).* New York: Aldine De Gruyter.

Scott, Brent A. & Judge, Timothy A. 2006. "Insomnia, Emotions, and Job Satisfaction." *Journal of Management* 32 (5): 622-645.

Scurlock-Durana, Suzanne. 2010. *Full Body Presence: Learning to Listen to Your Body's Wisdom.* Novato, California: Nataraj Publishing.

Shapiro, Debbie. 2005. *Your Body Speaks Your Mind: Decoding the Emotional, Psychological, and Spiritual Messages that Underlie Illness.* Boulder: Sounds True.

Siegenthaler, K.L. 1997. "Health Benefits of Leisure." *Parks and Recreation* 32 (1): 24-31.

Spencer, Liz & Pahl, Ray. 2006. *Rethinking Friendship: Hidden Solidarities Today.* Princeton, New Jersey: Princeton University Press.

Stellar, J.E., Manzo, V.M., & Keltner, D. 2012. "Class and Compassion: Socioeconomic Factors Predict Responses to Suffering." *Emotion* 12(3): 449-59.

Steinbeck, John. 2002. *Travels with Charley in Search of America.* New York: Penguin Books.

Strauss-Blasche, G. Ekmekcioglu, C, & Markti, W. 2000. "Does vacation enable recuperation? Changes in well-being associated with time away from work." *Occupational Medicine* 50 (3): 167-172.

Tacey D. 2004. *The Spirituality Revolution: The Emergence of Contemporary Spirituality.* New York: Brunner Routledge.

Twist, Lynne. 2003. *The Soul of Money: Reclaiming the Wealth of our Inner Resources.* New York: W.W. Norton & Company.

Umberson, Debra. 2006. "Bad Marriage May Make You Sick." *Journal of Health and Social Behavior* 47: 1-16.

Vallerand. R.J. & Ratelle, C.F. 2002. "Intrinsic and Extrinsic Motivation: A Hierarchical Model." In *The Motivation and Self-Determination of Behavior: Theoretical and Applied Issues,* edited by E. L., Deci and R.M. Ryan. Rochester, NY: University of Rochester Press.

Walsh, R. 1999. *Essential Spirituality: Exercises from the World's Religions to Cultivate Kindness, Love, Joy, Peace, Vision, Wisdom, and Generosity.* New York: John Wiley & Sons, Inc.

World Health Organization. "Questions and Answers on Environmental Health." http://www.who.int/.

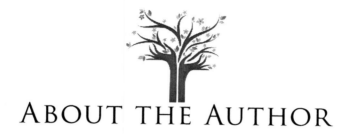

About the Author

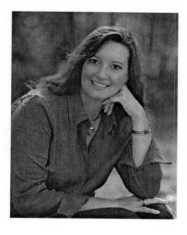

Katherine T. Kelly, Ph.D., M.S.P.H. is a pioneer of holistic and spiritual health, teaching her *Soul Health Model* throughout the country. She was the Director of Behavioral Science in Family Medicine at Wake Forest University, trained with the Mind-Body Medical Institute of Harvard University, and has owned her own holistic health and wellness center.

With over 23 years of direct client experience, Dr. Kelly doesn't just believe in helping patients to heal; instead, her mission is to help them to *evolve*. Using her own integrative framework—the *"Soul Health Model"*—Dr. Kelly approaches her work with clients from a "psycho-spiritual" perspective. She currently lives in Winston-Salem, North Carolina.

CPSIA information can be obtained
at www.ICGtesting.com
Printed in the USA
LVOW10s1641281116

514774LV00002B/522/P